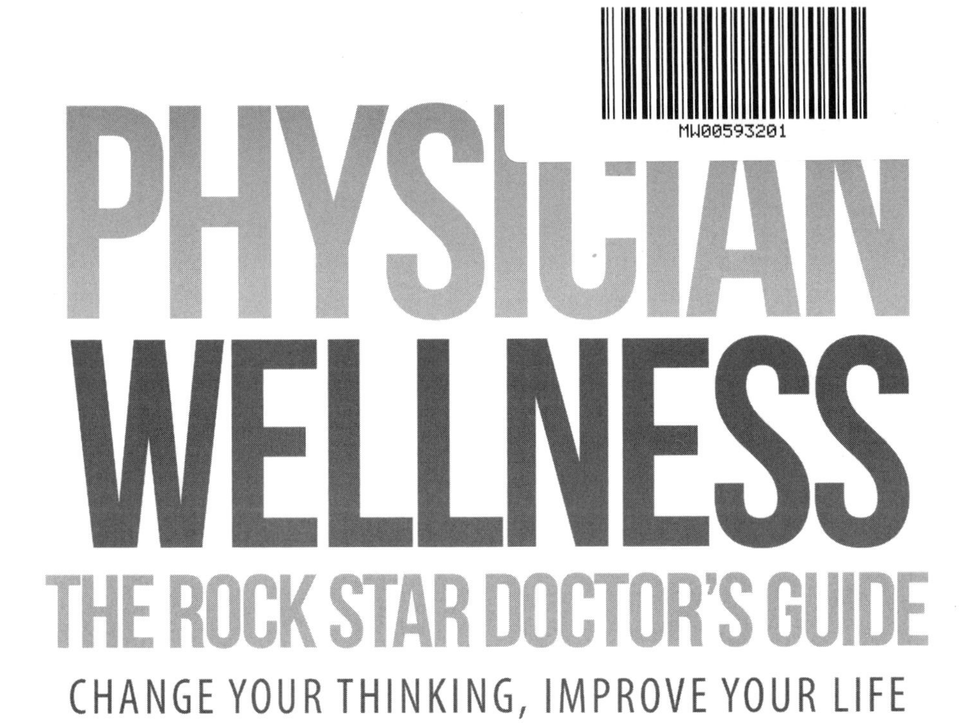

PHYSICIAN WELLNESS

THE ROCK STAR DOCTOR'S GUIDE

CHANGE YOUR THINKING, IMPROVE YOUR LIFE

REBEKAH BERNARD, MD
STEVEN COHEN, PsyD

PHYSICIAN WELLNESS: THE ROCK STAR DOCTOR'S GUIDE

CHANGE YOUR THINKING, IMPROVE YOUR LIFE

by Rebekah Bernard, MD and Steven Cohen, PsyD

AUTHORS' NOTE: The authors are not engaged in rendering professional advice or services to the individual reader. The ideas, suggestions, and exercises contained in the book are not intended as a substitute for consulting with your personal physician or psychologist. All matters regarding your health require medical supervision. Neither the author nor the publisher shall be liable or responsible for any loss or damage allegedly arising from any information of suggestion in this book.

While the authors have made every effort to provide accurate internet addresses and other contact information at the time of publication, neither the publisher nor the authors assume any responsibility for errors or changes that occur after publication. Further, the publisher does not have any control over and does not assume any responsibility for author or third-party websites or their content.

Book Layout and Cover Design: www.PearCreative.ca

ISBN Print: 978-0-9964509-3-5
ISBN eBook: 978-0-9964509-2-8

To Juan, Elisha, and Evan for promoting our wellness throughout this process and for being supportive despite the hours that we spent away from you while writing this book.

PSYCHOLOGY RULES

1. The system is broken. You don't have to be.
2. Stop catastrophizing.
3. Learn to stop procrastinating—today.
4. Find your intrinsic motivation.
5. Develop and maintain personal hobbies outside of medicine
6. Boundaries are your friend.
7. 'No' is a complete sentence.
8. The doctor should not be working harder than the patient.
9. People who really need to see a psychologist usually won't go. That's why the rest of us have to.
10. The better you take care of yourself, the better you can care for others

CONTENTS

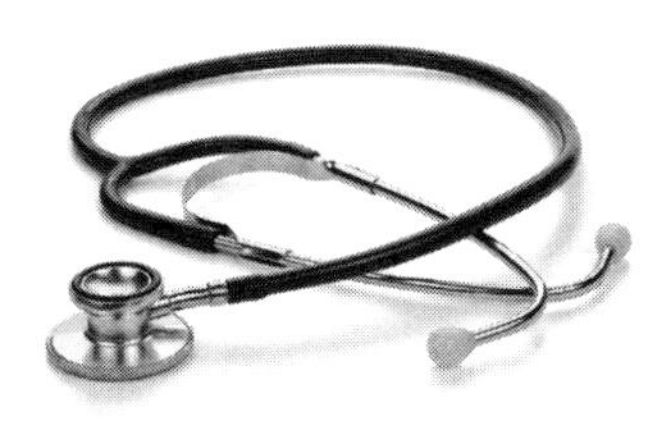

CHAPTER ONE

PHYSICIAN WELLNESS—WHAT MAKES THIS BOOK DIFFERENT?

If you've picked up this book, there is a reason. It means that you have the courage to take steps to improve your life and your career.

It's a tough time to be a physician. With the steadily growing demands and ever-waning rewards of our current health care system, doctors have become increasingly miserable, burned out, and depressed. And many physicians have simply had enough. In fact, nearly half of all doctors report that they are actively making plans to leave the clinical practice of medicine.[i]

While attention is beginning to be paid to the increasing strain on physicians, most expert recommendations for improving wellness rely heavily on organizational change. Unfortunately, individual doctors have little to no control over how their organizations function. And, when physician-specific advice is given, it tends to be well-meaning but vague—like recommending that doctors prioritize self-care and find work-life balance, without elaborating on how to achieve such a feat.

That's where this book is different.

Physician Wellness: The Rock Star Doctor's Guide will start you on a journey of using the science of psychology to overcome the challenges that each of us face as practicing physicians. By learning to think differently, you will acquire the tools that can help you to take back control of your personal life and your medical practice.

What you will not find in this book: Generic, one-size-fits-all recommendations intended just to get you through another day.

Instead, the physician will discover specific, practical, data-driven advice that you can apply to improve your everyday life and to help you make changes that deliver long term benefits.

Be warned: this book will not be easy. It's going to force you to develop a sense of self-awareness that can sometimes be uncomfortable. We will ask you to explore inner aspects of yourself as well as emotions that we often avoid acknowledging. That includes our own weaknesses and insecurities.

But we believe that the trade-off is well worth it because this book will help you to gain the insight and confidence to take charge of your life.

Each section also includes cognitive exercises (ROCK STAR ACTIVITIES) designed to reinforce your new skills and improve your results.

HOW TO USE THIS BOOK

Don't be daunted!

It's not necessary to read this book cover-to-cover or do every single exercise to be successful.

This book is meant to be a guide and a tool for your personal growth.

You can choose to read the entire book, or you can pick and choose the chapters that you feel will be most beneficial for your needs. Or, you can read it systematically, chapter by chapter, and take the time to process and practice each new skill before you move on to the next.

Again, you don't have to do it all! Even if you take away one or two new strategies, this book will change your life.

Why psychology?

The bottom line is that psychology works—numerous studies have shown that by learning to think differently, you can change not only how you feel, but also how you behave.[ii iii iv] And, by changing how you behave, you may positively influence the behavior of those around you.[v]

So, while some of the challenges in medicine may seem insurmountable, the simple act of thinking differently can improve how you cope with the problems in our health care system. Or, by thinking about your situation differently, you may find yourself empowered to make a bigger life change, such as switching jobs or even *"opting out"* of the traditional health care system and into an alternate medical practice.

How can this book help me?

One of the best ways to change your thinking is through cognitive behavioral therapy, or psychotherapy, usually with an experienced psychologist. But for many doctors, working with a psychologist isn't an option—we may not be ready or able to start our own individual psychotherapy at this stage in our lives. Consider this book as the next best option: A preliminary step toward using the techniques of psychology to ease the stressors that you face as a physician.

While we encourage every physician confronting emotional challenges to seek professional psychological counseling, we hope that this book will help you to begin healing and will motivate you to encourage others to get the help that they need. We also hope to inspire an ongoing discussion about how psychology can help with mental strain while removing the stigma of seeking treatment, something that comes too late for some physicians.

WHY IS THIS BOOK SO IMPORTANT? A PERSONAL MESSAGE

This book was inspired by the sudden death of a beloved community physician, someone that Dr. Rebekah Bernard, one of the authors of this book, had known and worked with for fifteen years. Here are her words:

When I first learned of this physician's death, I was shocked and deeply saddened—after all, he was only in his early 50s. But my shock turned to horror when murmurings from colleagues reached me—while his family had listed "natural causes" as the cause of death to avoid negative publicity, the physician had actually died of suicide.

How could this have happened? I reflected on my many years of friendship with this physician. I remembered how I often ran into him at doctor events and he always seemed so happy-go-lucky. I recalled the way I used to joke with him about how he seemed to be able to "do it all," working in the hospital and office, while giving lectures and participating in many committees and groups.

My heart broke to think that this physician, who gave so much to his patients, the community, and his colleagues, was silently suffering to the point where he felt that the best solution was to take his own life. And this physician was not alone. Around the same time that our county lost a beloved doctor, the county just north of us also lost a physician to suicide. And across our country, other physicians are suffering, with an estimated 400 doctors dying by suicide each year.[vi]

Physicians are experiencing increased emotional strain, often due to the burdens associated with the practice of modern medicine.[vii] I realized that something had to change. While we may not be able to change our system, ***we can change ourselves and our thinking using psychology.*** Fortunately, I happened to know just the right psychologist, Dr. Steven Cohen, to get this message out.

Together, we collaborated to write this book to explain how you can use psychological techniques to improve your thinking and your life. His advice throughout this book will serve as a guide and a starting point to the healing process that many physicians so desperately need.

As a physician, I have personally benefited from the use of psychology—unfortunately, it took me ten years in practice to realize that I could (and should) get help. Only when I faced an existential crisis of burnout in my own life did I begin to apply psychology to take control of my own personal and professional life. In fact, some of the clinical vignettes you will read in this book (every one of them true stories) are from my own painful experiences as a physician.

Once I began to use psychology techniques in my day-to-day interactions with patients and with those around me, I saw tremendous results that inspired me to learn more. And the light at the end of the tunnel is real—after fourteen years of being owned by various corporate entities I finally had the courage to open my own practice. Within a year, the practice was full, and by two years, I was able to add a physician partner.

Despite all the positive changes in my life, I still use psychological techniques to stay at my best. After all, there will always be difficult patients and life will continue to throw curve balls. Even Rock Star Doctors can benefit from psychology!

SO, WHAT IS A ROCK STAR DOCTOR, ANYWAY?

In 2015 I published "How to Be a Rock Star Doctor: The Complete Guide to Taking Back Control of Your Life and Your Profession." I had spent the last thirteen years as the most "productive" physician in settings as opposite as you can get from one other—a Federally Qualified Rural Health Center and a for-profit hospital-owned practice.

So, when my colleagues asked me for tips on how to see more patients while maintaining high patient satisfaction, I began sharing the handouts and forms and workarounds I had created to optimize my efficiency—and from that, *How to Be a Rock Star Doctor* was born.

A Rock Star Doctor is a physician who is beloved by patients, has a busy and thriving practice, and manages the office with the utmost efficiency. The Rock Star Doctor achieves this by knowing how to demonstrate the qualities that the patient considers to be the most important in a physician, and by using shortcuts and time-saving techniques whenever possible.

But there is a danger to being a Rock Star: The risk of burning out.

When you are a Rock Star Doctor, you are in demand. Patients want to see you—not only your current patients, but new patients. You acquire a waiting list and sometimes people get frustrated and angry that they can't get in to see you. You may feel guilty and bad that you can't accommodate everyone who wants to see you. And you are working longer hours than you may want.

As a Rock Star doctor, your employer values you, which brings benefits but also drawbacks. Your boss may constantly ask you to participate in committees and take leadership positions or let the new docs shadow you in clinic. When the CEO's kid is sick, naturally you are the first one they call. You start to feel frustrated and anxious, but it is hard to say no. You find yourself getting behind on your charts because you had to leave clinic early to attend another mindless meeting… again.

You see how the pressure can start to build, and the expectations that we put on ourselves intensify. And indeed, sometimes the higher we rise, the harder we fall. In fact, a Rock Star physician is at risk for the same issues that Rock Star celebrities face, including behavioral issues, poor financial decisions, alcohol and drug abuse, relationship problems, and depression and suicide.

So how does a Rock Star doctor prevent burnout? By using psychology.

WHAT IS PSYCHOLOGY, AND WHAT CAN IT DO FOR ME?

Psychology is the study of the human mind, and yes, it is a real science. We can use psychology to analyze our thought processes and beliefs, and to help us develop insight about our behavior. We all studied this stuff in med school. But very few physicians actually apply the principles of psychology to the working of our own minds—or to those around us.

The truth is, the way that we think about things, whether consciously or not, influences our actions. Understanding what drives us to think in a certain way can empower us to change aspects about our own behavior and even to influence the behavior of those around us. A solid base of scientific evidence shows that by changing the way that we think, using cognitive behavioral therapy (CBT), we can begin to change our behavioral patterns.[viii]

While the best way to delve into the nitty-gritty of our own psyche is by working with a personal psychologist, we can learn to apply basic psychology concepts on our own.

That's where this book comes in. By describing the various elements of cognitive behavioral therapy and giving you exercises to practice on your own, you can start the process of changing your thinking and changing your life.

HOW TO USE PSYCHOLOGY TO ADDRESS PHYSICIAN BURNOUT

Working in health care has become one of the most stressful occupations in the United States.While most professions in the US have reported decreased rates of burnout, the rate of physician burnout has skyrocketed, with more than 50% of doctors across all specialties reported feeling burned out in 2016.[xi]

Physicians in every specialty are reporting increasing levels of burnout. And, studies show that women have about double the rates of their male colleagues,[x] with the very highest levels of burnout being seen among women working in more traditionally male-dominated fields like urology, orthopedic surgery, critical care, and cardiology.[xi]

What is burnout? *(*Author's note: We recognize that the word "burnout" has gained a negative connotation for many, and we do prefer to focus on physician wellness. However, we have decided to use the term to be consistent with the vocabulary used in the scientific literature cited throughout this text.)*

Burnout is characterized by three major symptoms:

- Exhaustion, with a loss of enthusiasm for work
- Depersonalization and cynicism, (think TV's *Dr. House*) with a tendency towards seeing patients less as people but rather as objects or barriers to your own needs
- Reduced sense of personal accomplishment or a sense that work is no longer meaningful, more commonly seen in women physicians than in men[xii]

Burnout is a huge problem because it leads to physician distress, including depression, anxiety, and increased use of alcohol and substances as a form of self-medication. Because burned out physicians are prone to poor impulse control and impaired judgment, they can get themselves into trouble at work and home. And, burned out doctors are getting out of medicine because they have had enough.

WHY IS PHYSICIAN BURNOUT INCREASING?

Medicine is a field that requires an enormous output of energy from clinicians. The physical demands of prolonged hours and overnight shifts, as well as the emotional drain of working with scores of hurting and needy patients day in and day out takes a toll on physicians. Since the medical profession has always been known for its physical and emotional demands, why is burnout now getting so much worse?

Loss of autonomy and control

As the culture of health care has transitioned from a doctor-in-charge to an administrator-in-charge model, physicians increasingly face a loss of autonomy and control in the day-to-day practice of medicine.

Part of this loss of control is unintentionally our own fault. In medical school and residency, we were trained to care for patients, and learned very little about business and health care management. And since most of us just want to take care of patients rather than handle the business end of medicine, we have turned our backs on anything that doesn't relate directly to patient care, trusting others to manage the non-clinical aspects of running a practice.

As the burden of mandates imposed by governmental agencies and insurance payers has grown, we have increasingly turned towards group practices and hospital employment to save us from administrative headaches so we could focus on patient care.

Physicians are notoriously resilient. We're also famous people-pleasers. So, when our practice managers asked us to do a little extra, to click a few more boxes, to be a bit more flexible with a new electronic health record or perhaps to adapt our systems and practices to improve reimbursement, we've just nodded our heads and rolled with the program. We're resilient like that.

But before we knew it, doctors were working for practice managers rather than for patients. Suddenly we found ourselves spending more time on paperwork and computers than being face-to-face with patients. Worse, our administrators had become our captors rather than our helpers.

No wonder physicians feel increasingly powerless and frustrated. We bear the ultimate responsibility for patient outcomes. But we have lost control over how we practice medicine each day in many of our work environments.

The bottom line is that the health care system is broken. The good news is that you don't have to be.

PSYCHOLOGY RULE #1:

The system is broken. You don't have to be.

Fortunately, no matter how bad a situation is, you can almost always do something to change your perspective or create an alternative. Depending on where you are in your phase of life, your solution might range from learning to cope with the pressures at work by using positive thinking and efficiency techniques, to leaving your job for another opportunity—or to a completely radical change like opening your own third-party free office. Always remember that no matter how bad things seem, you always have options.

PSYCHOLOGY TIP

Remember that no matter how bad things seem, you always have options.

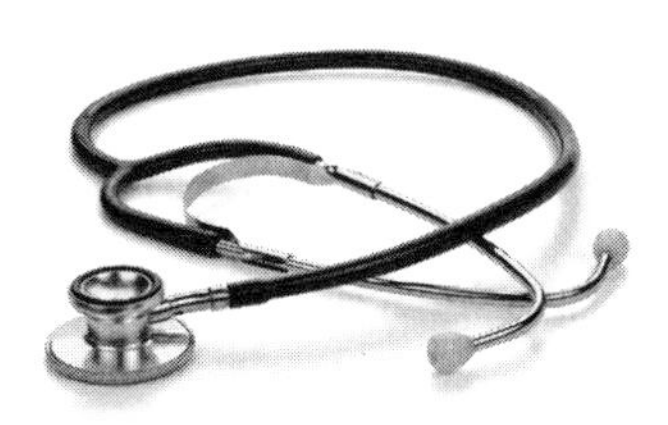

CHAPTER TWO

LEARNING HOW TO THINK DIFFERENTLY

"No problem can withstand the assault of sustained thinking."
- Voltaire

We are always thinking. Always. Our brain is a little nonstop engine constantly firing synapses, whether we want it to or not. Consider how active our mind is when we are sleeping. Think about how we dream in such vivid and creative detail that we can't even imagine during our waking hours.

Unfortunately, much of our thinking is neither directed nor sustained. And, it is easy for our thinking to go wrong, or in psychology terms, to become maladaptive. This is how cognitive behavioral therapy (CBT) can really help.

CBT is the process of identifying and correcting wrong or faulty thinking patterns, termed *"cognitive distortions."*

PSYCHOLOGY TIP

A cognitive distortion is an inaccurate or illogical thought process.

Some of the more common types of cognitive distortions described by David Burns in *The Feeling Good Handbook (1989)*,[xiii] include;

- Emotional reasoning, or "I feel something, therefore it must be true"
- Jumping to conclusions, without real evidence
- Filtering, or ignoring everything good about your day and only focusing on the bad, even when you have lots of good things in your life
- Personalization, or assuming that everything you do has a tremendous impact on others, even when there is no clear or obvious link
- Catastrophizing (see chapter 3)

CLINICAL VIGNETTE

A retired internist described a great example of the cognitive distortion of "personalization" in medicine. *"I had just started a farmer on statin therapy for high cholesterol. A week later he came in with severe rhabdomyolysis. I immediately thought 'Oh my God, I've killed him.' I admitted him to the hospital, started pumping him full of fluids, and was just tortured by the thought that he might die from the medicine I had given him. A few hours later his wife came by the hospital and said, 'Doc, do you think this has anything to do with him getting struck by lightning out in the field yesterday? I told him we should call 911 but he said he was just going to go see you at the office the next day.'"*

Once you learn how to identify a faulty thought process, CBT focuses on discovering an alternate way of thinking which you then practice until the healthier way of thinking comes more naturally. This is called *"cognitive reframing."*

PSYCHOLOGY TIP

Cognitive reframing is the process of identifying and then challenging a faulty/ illogical thought or emotion, and then practicing seeing a more positive alternative.

HOW TO CHANGE YOUR THINKING

The best way to improve your thinking is to work with a psychologist trained in CBT. However, several self-directed techniques can be helpful.

Learn to recognize distorted/irrational thoughts and feelings

The first step in cognitive reframing is to learn to recognize faulty thoughts and feelings. One sign of unhealthy thinking is that it tends to be intrusive and repetitive—the thought or feeling pushes to the forefront of your mind and distracts you from other activities. We may find ourselves thinking these thoughts repeatedly without meaning to.

Another sign of distorted thinking is that these thoughts are usually illogical and not reality-based. They tend towards extremes of "always" and "never" or "black" and "white." Distorted thinking is so powerful that even when all evidence points to the contrary, and everyone around is pointing out a fact, the person will still believe their incorrect thought over what the reality that rest of the world is sharing with them.

CLINICAL VIGNETTE

Dr. E battled an eating disorder since her teenage years. She worked very hard on the cognitive distortion of body dysmorphia—even when she was excessively thin and family members expressed concern for her near-skeletal frame, she still "saw" herself as overweight.

Signs of distorted thoughts and feelings:

- Intrusive/ distracting
- Repetitive
- Illogical/ not reality-based
- Extremes (always/never, black/white)

Any time you have a distorted thought or emotion, the first step is to acknowledge that thought. Many physicians get caught up in the "why" of the thought/ feeling—*"why do I feel this way?"* Asking why is not helpful. Instead, simply acknowledge what you think or feel. *"I feel very anxious about the meeting I have tomorrow. I am worried that I am going to get fired."*

Challenge the distorted thought/ feeling

The next step in cognitive reframing is to intellectually and logically challenge the distorted belief. Ask yourself:

- Is there any proof that these thoughts are valid?
- Is this belief based on reality or facts?
- What evidence do I have to support this belief?

Practice cognitive reframing

If you have challenged your beliefs and found that they are indeed illogical—there is no proof or evidence that they are true—then the next step is to consider alternative explanations for your belief—in other words, reframe the situation. *"My boss may want to invite me to be on a committee. I've been doing a great job lately, so maybe I'm getting a promotion."*

PSYCHOLOGY TIP

Acknowledge your distorted thoughts/ emotions. Logically challenge your beliefs and consider alternative explanations.

Remember that thoughts and feelings are not facts. We can train ourselves to accept this reality through cognitive reframing, an important part of CBT. In fact, functional imaging MRI studies have shown that the use of cognitive therapy changes our neural pathways from the emotional to the analytical. It re-wires our brain circuitry and blocks the vicious cycle of intrusive thinking.[xiv]

PSYCHOLOGY TIP

Cognitive reframing can help to rewire brain circuit pathways so that our thinking transforms from emotional to analytical.

ROCK STAR ACTIVITY

Practice cognitive reframing using the following worksheet.

If you experience an incident that causes you worry thoughts, practice cognitive reframing using the following chart. First, label the emotion that you are feeling. Then, list the automatic thoughts that you find yourself experiencing, and ask yourself how much you believe those thoughts on a scale of 1-10.

Now, deliberately reframe the automatic thought by replacing it with an alternate, likely explanation that is positive. Rate how much you believe the reframed thought on a scale of 1-10.

Review the example scenario, and then try it yourself.

Example scenario: You find out a patient of yours died unexpectedly from a brain aneurysm. You just saw him the office one week earlier for an ear infection.

Emotion	Automatic thoughts:	How much do you believe this? (1-10)	Reframe the automatic thought:	How much do I believe the reframe? (1-10)
Guilty	"I must have missed something. I could have prevented this."	9	"I provided the same degree of care I always provide and treated the concerns that presented. There is nothing I would have done differently if I were in that same scenario again."	5
Anxious	"I'm going to do this again. I am a bad doctor."	8.5	"There were no signs to have indicated an aneurysm in this patient. I cannot predict the future and one case does not define my overall abilities."	9
Scared	"I'm going to get sued and lose my medical license."	9	"I know I did everything correctly, and the family even contacted me to tell me what happened and thanked me for all I did for the patient. There is nothing to suggest that they blame me and there is nothing that would affect my license."	10

SCENARIO:

Emotion	Automatic thoughts:	How much do you believe this? (1-10)	Reframe the automatic thought:	How much do I believe the reframe? (1-10)

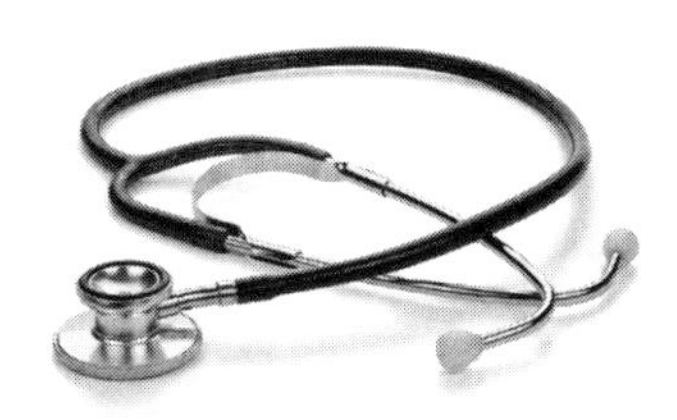

CHAPTER THREE

STOP CATASTROPHIZING

Catastrophizing is an important cognitive distortion that often affects physicians, perhaps because our training encourages us to "think of the worst" when evaluating our patients to avoid missing a serious diagnosis. Catastrophizing occurs when we assume the worst will happen and, indeed, see all possible outcomes to a situation as being a worst-case scenario.

CLINICAL VIGNETTE

Dr. B was a 35-year old physician in the depth of the great recession. Her husband of 5-years had lost his job and was emotionally unsupportive. She felt trapped by an overpriced house which was purchased during the housing bubble. She despised her job at an RVU-factory so much that she couldn't fall asleep at night for dread of waking up the next day to go to work. One night she called her sister in despair, who said: *"If you hate your job, quit."* But what about the house? The mortgage? *"Let it foreclose. File for bankruptcy. Divorce your husband. Move in with me and get a job working locum tenens. Would that be the end of the world?"* Dr. B suddenly realized that she wasn't trapped. She had choices. This changed her outlook and although she didn't take her sister's recommendations, she did later leave her job (and her husband) for a happier situation.

Elements of catastrophic thinking include:

- Rumination, or replaying a potentially adverse scenario in our mind, like imagining a bad conversation with your boss in extensive detail.
- Magnification, or making a situation greater than it really is—a notice that the company is making some cutbacks immediately convinces you that you are going to lose your job.
- Helplessness, or the thought that there is absolutely nothing that you can do to change these horrific outcomes, and therefore there is no reason to try.

CLINICAL VIGNETTE

A patient of mine gave me the perfect example of catastrophic thinking recently. She was having gynecologic symptoms, which turned out to be a simple yeast infection, quickly resolved with one tablet of an antifungal pill. However, prior to seeing me, she had convinced herself that she had a sexually transmitted disease (despite a monogamous relationship) which would render her infertile, causing her husband to leave her and she would die alone. Talk about catastrophizing!

To avoid catastrophizing, you must:

1. Identify the distorted thinking pattern of rumination and magnification, especially when the thoughts are unrealistic and

illogical.

2. Challenge the belief by asking yourself: "Is this belief based on fact?"
3. Reframe the situation. Once you have identified the cognitive distortion, you can make a deliberate effort to reframe the situation in a positive light by contemplating an alternate scenario.

For example, you receive a subpoena demanding your appearance in court. Your first thought is: *"I'm getting sued."* You instantly go into panic mode, imagining blocking your schedule for days at a time, sitting on the stand being grilled by a prosecutor, and losing your entire assets to a lawsuit.

Stop, close your eyes, and deliberately imagine a positive, alternate outcome, such as: Calling the attorney's office to inquire and learning that they only need medical records. Visualize yourself on the phone, calm and controlled, inquiring about the nature of the subpoena. The attorney tells you that you don't even have to testify—it was a blanket subpoena and all they need from you are records.

You can do this for any type of situation in which you feel a sense of overwhelming helplessness and doom or despair. If a recurrent catastrophic thought pops into your head, stop, close your eyes, and repeat the positive scenario again. You may have to do this repeatedly until you retrain your brain patterns.

Stop practicing wrong thinking

Envisioning positive outcomes takes practice and work. The problem is that we unintentionally practice thinking incorrectly about things all the time. For example, if we are dreading our upcoming board examination, we may spend weeks leading up to the exam worrying about the test, thinking about how hard it will be, imagining ourselves sweating over impossible test questions, and pondering the consequences of failure. This type of thinking intrudes on our ability to study and learn. By the time we take the exam, we have worked ourselves into a state of panic that negatively impacts our test-taking ability.

Instead, we should deliberately imagine ourselves in a clear, focused, and positive frame of mind as we study for the test. Then, when we sit down to take the exam, we feel calm and confident. We open the exam booklet. And right away, we know the answer to the first question! Visualize yourself bubbling in or clicking the correct answer and moving on to the next question. Again, you know the answer! You've got this! Now think about getting your test results and seeing your passing result. You feel great. You worked hard, and you earned it.

The key to this successful approach is to think positive thoughts—not to avoid negative ones. For example, if you are playing golf and you take a few practice swings, the last thing you want to tell yourself is: "Don't slice it, don't slice it!" If you focus on not slicing, what are you sure to do? Why, slice, of course! Instead, you want to focus on what you want to achieve—imagine yourself hitting a nice, straight, even shot.

The more you exercise positive thinking, the better you can cope with negative events. That in turn, reduces overall anxiety.

PSYCHOLOGY TIP

Practice thinking the way you want to think and stop practicing wrong thinking!

Ask yourself: would this be a real catastrophe or merely undesirable?

Another way to cope with catastrophic thinking is to practice distinguishing between merely unpleasant outcomes and catastrophes. While getting fired would be very unpleasant, it wouldn't be a catastrophe—you are very likely to be able to find another job, and who knows, it might even be better than the one you lost. Losing your medical license? Now that might be a catastrophe. Or would it? You could always get a job teaching high school biology. Well, maybe catastrophe is the right word after all.

Play the script to the end

Another technique for managing anxious thoughts and catastrophic thinking is to consider playing the script out to the end. What is the actual worst-case scenario that could happen, and what would life be like in that scenario? You get fired from your job. What does that look like? You find another job. Maybe you must take out a loan to cover your bills in the meantime. Or worse, you file for bankruptcy like millions of Americans do each year. Maybe you move in to your parents' basement. The bottom line? You didn't die. You survived. You will recover. Maybe you will even come out better.

PSYCHOLOGY RULE #2

Stop catastrophizing.

ROCK STAR ACTIVITY

Practice correct thinking using the following worksheet.

When you identify a self-defeating thought, ask yourself three questions to determine if the thought is rational. Acknowledge the incorrect thought and decide not to think that way any longer. Identify a new, rational/positive belief and practice correct thinking.

EXAMPLE:

Identify a self-defeating thought.
"I have my boards next week and I am going to fail them."

Now, ask yourself these questions:

Is there any proof that these thoughts are valid? __Yes__x__No
("I cannot predict the future to know whether I will pass or fail.")

Is this belief based on reality or fact? __Yes__x__No
("I have not taken the Boards yet, so I don't know how I will do."

Do I have any evidence to support this belief? __x__Yes__No
("I haven't passed any of the practice exams.")

If the answer is 'no' to any of these questions, then you know that this belief is irrational. Next:

1. Acknowledge the thought and choose not to think that way any longer.
("I am afraid I am going to fail the Boards and this will affect my ability to practice.")

2. Identify a new, rational or positive belief:
"I have been practicing and studying and the more I continue to practice the more likely it will be that I can pass this test because I know my stuff."

3. Practice thinking the new belief
(imagine yourself taking the Boards confident and prepared; visualize yourself getting your results and the way you feel as you see that passing score, the emotions you experience in that

moment)—this may be difficult to imagine at first, but the more you practice, the better you will get!

NOW, TRY IT YOURSELF!

Identify the self-defeating thought:

____

____

____

Now, ask yourself these questions:

Is there any proof that these thoughts are valid? __Yes__No

Is this belief based on reality or fact? __Yes__No

Do I have any evidence to support this belief? __Yes__No

If the answer is 'no' to any of these questions, then you know that this belief is irrational. Next:

1. Acknowledge the thought and choose not to think that way any longer

2. Identify a new, rationale or positive belief:

____

____

____

3. Practice thinking the new belief

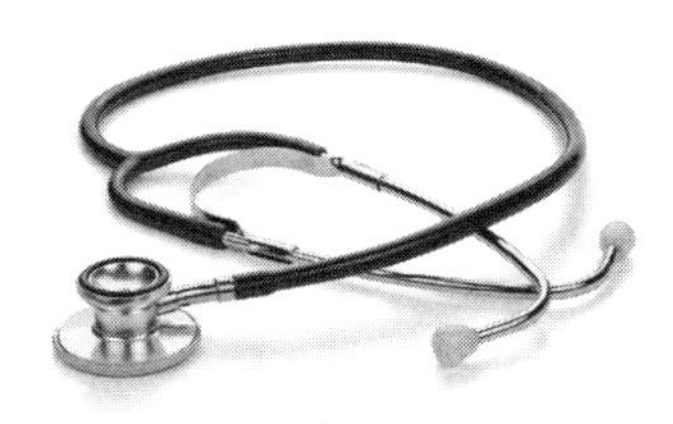

CHAPTER FOUR

MINDFULNESS, MEDITATION AND MENTAL REST

I know, I know, we promised no touchy-feely stuff, but it's simply impossible to ignore the importance of mindfulness and its impact on our health and well-being.

Mindfulness and meditation have been shown to improve wellness, but the problem is that we aren't sure of the very best way to do it—there just isn't enough rigorous scientific study on the topic.[xv] One thing that is definite is that our brains do need a rest from the constant bombardment and stimulation from the outside world. In other words, allow your mind the opportunity for "constructive internal reflection."[xvi]

Have you ever had an epiphany? You can call it a lightbulb moment, an "A-ha moment" a la Oprah Winfrey, or a revelation. But, suddenly and seemingly out of the blue, a thought crystallizes in your mind. Suddenly, the solution to a problem or issue in your life suddenly becomes apparent. Usually, this epiphany is something that your working mind never saw coming. But once it occurs, the answer is obvious and can be life-changing.

Usually those epiphanies occur when the mind is in a non-distracted state. Think of Euripides relaxing in his bath, as the solution for buoyancy occurs to him. Eureka! Or Isaac Newton, dawdling under an apple tree as the theory of gravity strikes him. Tesla was known for taking long rambling walks and would rush home to jot down the ideas that popped into his mind—just little things, like, say the creation of electricity.

Often my best ideas occur to me when I am getting out of the shower, drying my hair, or just about to fall asleep at night. Why? Because these are the few times that I am just letting my mind wander without outside stimuli. No radio blaring the latest political scandal, no Facebook feed, no fictional television drama to distract my brain from its most important job—thinking.

We need to take some time to just let our brain do its work, uninterrupted. You can choose to do this in the form of meditation, through the practice of mindfulness, or following the example of Albert Einstein who like Nicolai Tesla was known for taking daily walks. Or you can just let your mind wander while you are doing something mundane like housework, taking a shower, or walking the dogs. The key is to minimize outside noise and interruptions—let your mind ramble without being distracted by music or TV. It will feel eerily silent at first, but then you may be able to start to hear your own thoughts.

Simply put, mindfulness is a process of deliberately keeping your thoughts and your focus in the moment.

Mindfulness can be as simple as going for a walk and taking note of the color of the sky, the feel of the breeze on your face, the smell of freshly cut grass—while gently pushing any external thoughts outside of the moment out of your mind. It can be sitting quietly for two minutes and breathing slowly in and out, while focusing on your breathing. It can occur in a yoga class. Or it can be done as a body scan, also known as progressive muscle relaxation (see ROCK STAR ACTIVITY).

There are a multitude of books, websites, and apps to help you with mindfulness and meditation, included in the resources at the end of the book.

Gratitude

Taking a few minutes to think about the things you are grateful for can improve your mood and outlook.[xvii] Some studies have even shown that people who practiced gratitude by keeping a gratitude journal had improved health.[xviii] Even if the only thing you can think of now is indoor plumbing, write it down and think about what life would be like without it. You'll feel happier!

Narrative Medicine

Sharing your feelings reduces stress. The Mayo clinic showed this—just giving doctors an hour together every other week to talk about their stressors lowered their levels of burnout.[xix] Try to schedule lunch or even coffee with friends and colleagues every week or two. Then just vent about life. It helps.

If you can't meet face-to-face, consider creating a virtual network. Send a group text or email to your residency or med school buddies, or form a social media group for your colleagues.

Another option is to join an existing virtual group—social media sites and listservs allow like-minded physicians of all different specialties and interests to gather online, posting messages and comments about a variety of topics.

In addition to talking with friends and colleagues, journaling can help you to take note of your moods and thoughts, which you can later analyze for patterns and triggers. Keep in mind that when you are journaling, you don't have to write in complete sentences—a big reason why some people avoid journaling. Shorthand and scribbling is just fine.

Journals are also a great place to write down ideas and epiphanies that occur to you—when a thought pops into your head, write it down immediately! As much as you promise yourself, you won't remember it later.

ROCK STAR ACTIVITY

Progressive muscle relaxation / body scan technique

To perform the body scan technique, lay down on a mat, close your eyes, and visualize your body, starting from your toes and moving up to the top of your head. As you visualize each part of the body, tense the muscle groups of that area, holding them as you inhale, and then releasing them on the exhalation. Continue to move upwards until your entire body is relaxed.

As an added challenge, try to see if you can limit yourself to only tensing one specific muscle while simultaneously keeping the other muscle groups as relaxed as possible.

ROCK STAR ACTIVITY

Gratitude journal

Start a gratitude journal. Write down five things for which you are appreciative. Reflect on what life would be if those things were not in your life. Try to do this daily.

1.____

2.____

3.____

4.____

5.____

ROCK STAR ACTIVITY

Narrative medicine

Talking about our feelings helps improve wellness. Pick one of the following and implement it this week:

- Schedule a time to meet with a colleague
- Write in a journal
- Join a virtual group

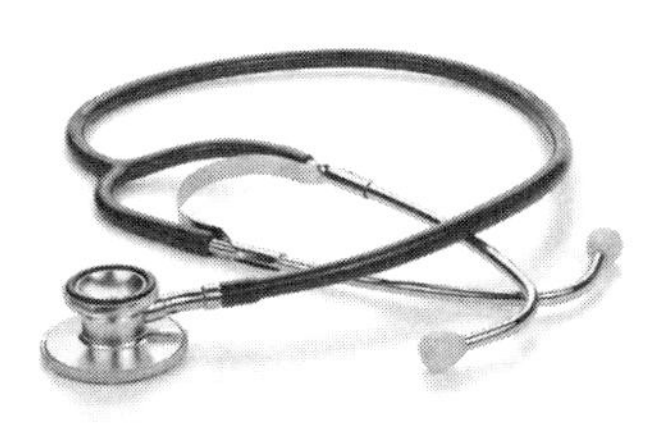

CHAPTER FIVE

USE PSYCHOLOGY TO MANAGE TIME AND AVOID PROCRASTINATION

There never seems to be enough time in the day to complete the ever-growing list of tasks that physicians need to accomplish. Doctors have been forced to become paper-pushers, now spending from half to two-thirds of their entire workday on paperwork. [xx]

The electronic record has much to do with this increase in documentation time. While we have always had plenty of paperwork to do, the nature of our work has changed drastically.

Back in the old days before electronic records, my desk would be stacked high with paper charts waiting to be reviewed, which in some ways was not necessarily a bad thing. I could see the mountain of work waiting, and so could everyone else. Routinely visitors would stop by my office to talk, visibly blanch as they took in the massive number of charts on my desk, and quickly offer to come back another time when I wasn't so overwhelmed.

Another benefit to paper charts was that I could see myself making a dent in the work to be done, as I sorted through and removed completed charts. And there was a sense of gratification from clearing my desk by the end of the day—or at least neatly re-stacking the work of lesser importance for tomorrow.

Times have changed. That mountain of paperwork is still there (and then some!). But now it lurks behind our computer screen in a variety of software programs that constantly demand our attention—in our electronic record, our patient portals, and our multiple email accounts. Since the work is hidden, no one else really empathizes with our plight. Since we don't appear visibly busy, it's no big deal for an administrator, nurse, or drug rep to stop and shoot the breeze.

Additionally, with electronic records, as soon as we click through to complete one task, another one pops up to take its place. The work never seems to end and there is never a sense of completion or accomplishment.

Is it any wonder that physicians often develop problems with procrastination?

Unfortunately, when we put off completing tasks like charting, our level of distress skyrockets. Understanding why we procrastinate and taking steps to change our thinking can help us reduce stress.

PSYCHOLOGY RULE #3

Learn to stop procrastinating—today.

WHY WE PROCRASTINATE

The most obvious reason for procrastination is simply because we don't want to do a task, or because we don't want to do the task *right at that moment*. The task may be tedious or emotionally painful. It may just get in the way of doing something enjoyable. Or, it may be that we don't have the time to finish the task if we start it now.

There are less obvious, but critical factors that lead to procrastination. One often unnoticed cause of procrastination is a lack of time awareness.

TIME AWARENESS

Time awareness is the ability to estimate how long a given task is going to take, along with the sense of time progressing as you are engaged in that task. While some people have an inherent natural ability of time awareness, others must work to acquire and develop this skill.

Think of the people in your life who are chronically late. Many of them often have little to no awareness of how tardy they are. We all know that person who regularly says: "I'll be there in 15 minutes," and when they show up in an hour and a half, they have no idea of the discrepancy. This tends to be a particular problem for people with attention deficit disorder, as they often have a very impaired ability to estimate time intervals.

People with poor time awareness skills struggle with procrastination because they have difficulty estimating how long it will take them to accomplish something. If you don't really know how long it truly takes you to do certain tasks—how long you spend in the exam room with patients, or how long it really takes to finish a note, or even how long it takes you to get from point A to point B, you run the risk of always being behind schedule.

The more you run behind, the more likely you will need to put something else off, like finishing charts, because you must move on to the next patient or go from the clinic to the hospital. The longer you put things off, the more they build up, and the more behind you get.

PSYCHOLOGY TIP

People with poor time awareness tend to be chronic procrastinators.

TECHNIQUES TO IMPROVE TIME AWARENESS

Time awareness is not something that everyone is inherently good at, but it can be learned. Start by getting a stopwatch or timer. Estimate how long you think it will take you to do a routine daily task, such as taking a shower. Write down your estimate. Then do the task with a stopwatch running. Once you have completed the task, click the stopwatch to stop the timer, but don't look at the timer yet!

Now, here is the key part of this exercise. Once you have finished whatever task you are doing, mentally estimate how long you think it took you to complete that task. Write down the number. Now, look at the watch and how long it actually took. The difference between those numbers tells you about your ability to perceive time.

The good news is that you can train yourself to improve your ability to sense time. As you practice estimating and then validating how long it takes you to perform daily activities, your perception will improve. Use the ROCK STAR ACTIVITY below as a guide to improve your time awareness skills.

Even if you are very good at knowing how long it takes *you* to do a task, it becomes more difficult when other people are factored into the equation. Practicing these exercises can help. In Chapter 10 we will use the time perception exercise again to help improve your efficiency in the exam room.

CONSIDER TRANSITION TIMES

One of the biggest problems with procrastination and time management is a failure to consider transition times into your planning. Transitions are times between activities—like getting from point A to point B for meetings or finishing office notes between patients.

By scheduling transition times into your day, using the same time awareness technique discussed above, your day will run more smoothly and on-time. For example, if you have an appointment scheduled at 1 PM, and another at 2 PM, ask yourself what time the 1 PM appointment will end, and if that gives you enough time to get to the next appointment. Without factoring in transition time, you will always feel rushed and frazzled as you run late.

MANAGING PROCRASTINATION BY SCHEDULING TASKS

One of the best ways to battle procrastination is to schedule tasks using specific time slots. Vague time descriptions ("I'll do it later/ tomorrow") don't work and worsen procrastination tendencies. Be sure to schedule precisely when to start and when to finish each task.

Keep a calendar and make a schedule of what you are going to accomplish that day. Make sure your goals are realistic.

For example, if you have thirty charts to complete but only have time to finish fifteen, then set your goal at fifteen.

This way, when you finish the fifteen charts, you experience a sense of accomplishment which fuels your intrinsic motivation to do more. If you had set your goal to thirty and then failed, only completing fifteen, your sense of failure reinforces procrastination. On the flip side, if you schedule fifteen and finish twenty, then you are a Rock Star!

In this same sense, scheduling more painful tasks for shorter intervals of time can help make them more palatable. It may seem futile to complete 10 charts when you have a hundred to do. However, by just getting something done, you are still putting a dent in your workload without causing yourself mental strain. Tell yourself: *"I am going to work on my charts for 30 minutes."* Once you are done, reflect on the effort you put in.

Think of it like setting off on a long car trip. If you have a thousand miles to your destination, you don't think, "999 more miles to go, 998 more miles, 997…" Rather, you take it in segments: "200 miles to the next stopping point," and so on.

ROCK STAR ACTIVITY

Time awareness study

Choose some simple activities and practice your time awareness. Start by pre-estimating how long you think it will take you to do something. Then, time yourself doing the activity, and before you check the timer, estimate how long you think it took. Now, look to see the actual time it took. The more you do this, the better you will get at perceiving time.

Example worksheet:

Activity	Pre-estimate of time it will take	Estimate of how long you think it took	Actual time it took
Take a shower	5 min	3 min	7 min
Walk one block			
Drive from the clinic to hospital			

NOW TRY IT YOURSELF:

Activity	Pre-estimate of time it will take	Estimate of how long you think it took	Actual time it took

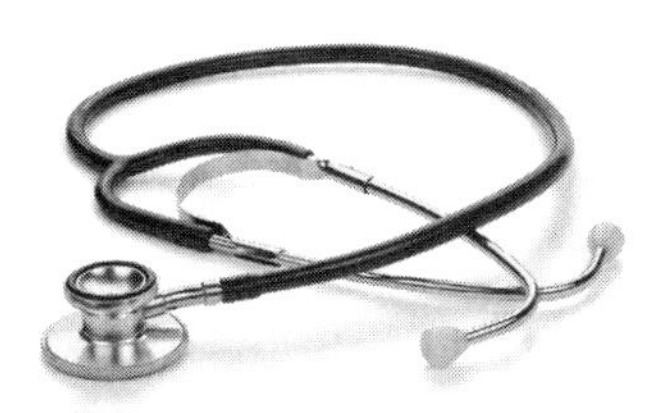

CHAPTER SIX

USE PSYCHOLOGY TO GET YOUR NOTES DONE

Medical record keeping or "charting" is one of the biggest sources of stress for physicians, particularly in the era of electronic health records. Most clinicians struggle with getting charts completed, with doctors now spending an average of one to two hours per day after work completing medical records. [xxi]

Often doctors have no control over which electronic health record their employer chooses, nor any input into making improvements to the system. That leads to plenty of frustration and anxiety.

Using computerized records also tends to trigger some of our insecurities and personality issues. For example, those of us who type our notes may fall prey to obsessive-compulsiveness, as we find ourselves editing, rewriting, and maybe even saving our notes to close "later" in case we missed something. Or, if we use templates that require shifting from one screen to another, our attention-deficit kicks in. Then we struggle to focus on the work that needs to be completed.

This constant expense of energy leads to anxiety and stress that may lead us to put off completing our notes. Psychology can help.

CLINICAL VIGNETTE

An internist with many medically complicated patients converted from paper records to an electronic health system. He is finding it hard to complete his notes because he worries about missing something. *"When I had paper charts, I knew where everything was. I could flip through the chart, keeping my finger on the current note, and then write down important information without losing my place. Now I worry I'm missing important details."* The internist has become anxious, is not completing his office notes because he is saving them to the end of the day to review without feeling the pressure of patients waiting for him. He stays at the office hours after the rest of the staff has gone home and is getting resentful.

Switching from paper records to computers requires a huge shift in routine. The procedures are completely different, requiring clinicians to learn an entirely different system from what they may have used for years. This requires a shift in the way we think about the patient visit and how we document information. And yet many organizations expect staff to "go live" on a brand-new system within days of its introduction.

It is important to remember that humans are creatures of habit and routine. Our brain is wired for patterns, and change can be perceived as a threat to be resisted. So, simply changing from one system to another won't be comfortable or easy. It's even worse when it is a radical change, such as transitioning between paper and computerized record keeping.

There is a tremendous learning curve involved—not only learning the new system-but also unlearning the way we did things before. For example, a major challenge to electronic systems is that it's almost too easy to make revisions to your notes. With paper and pen, if you wanted to change something in your note, you needed to draw a single line through the incorrect text, initial it, and then keep going. There was no going back to fix misspelled words, clarify context or make your words sound more eloquent. With a computer screen, you can spend unlimited amounts of time tweaking your note to be *"just right."* But who are we writing this note for, anyway?

DEALING WITH ANXIETY IN CHARTING

To defeat note-writing obsession, start by asking yourself: *"Who is going to benefit from this note?"*

PSYCHOLOGY TIP

Ask yourself when charting: "Who will benefit from this note?"

The medical record is primarily for yourself—to record your thinking at the time of the visit and your plan of action—and for other clinicians to understand your medical thinking. Of course, it can benefit you in the case of a malpractice suit to show your medical decision making. Finally, we must write our notes to benefit the payer—the insurance company or Medicare—to make sure that we have hit all the coding requirements to get paid for our services.

The common denominator is that none of these users' need or want to read a long soliloquy. They want only the important points. And, that's where bullet points come in.

ROCK STAR TIP

Bullet points are your friend.

Use bullet points to prevent obsessive-compulsive note writing

Don't waste time writing full sentences or long stories. Instead, use bullet points. This is particularly easy for documenting historical elements.

BEFORE BULLET POINTS:

Mrs. M is a 52-year-old woman with a past medical history of asthma presents with shortness of breath for three days, a cough productive of white sputum, tried Nyquil without relief. She has no fever or chills. She has had some wheezing.

AFTER BULLET POINTS:

- 52F, asthma
- SOB x 3 days
- Cough w/ white sputum
- Nyquil no relief
- No F/C + wheezing

Sure, the regular paragraph looks nice and neat. But I typed the bullet points in half the time. And any medical reader understands exactly what it means. Also, bullet points are easier for the eye to take in and read quickly.

MAKE TEMPLATES/ QUICK TEXTS

Templates (or macros, or quick texts) in the form of bullet points can be prepared in advance for many conditions. I have dozens of saved templates ranging from basic cold symptom advice to my work-up for chest pain to a generic pre-operative evaluation.

Using templates as a guide helps me to ensure that I don't forget an element of a particular work-up if I get distracted (*"by the way doctor, can you look at this rash…?*). They include my usual treatments for various conditions and document the advice that I routinely give patients. And they save me time from having to re-write the same information 20X/

day. I simply need to personalize and edit the template for the individual situation.

Although it may be hard to find the time to prepare these templates when you don't feel you have enough time as it is, they will save you far more time in the long run.

STOP OVER-ANALYZING YOUR NOTES

One of the biggest challenges for clinicians with obsessive-compulsive tendencies is the urge to analyze and re-analyze their notes. They often find it difficult to simply sign-off and close a note—*"what if I forgot to include something?"*

First, chances are that you didn't forget anything important, especially if you are getting your notes done close to the time of the visit. But, if you did forget something, you can always go back to the note and make an addendum after the fact.

Prove this to yourself by simply forcing yourself to CLOSE. THE. NOTE. That's it. Finish the note. Don't read it over. Simply sign it electronically and move on to the next task.

PSYCHOLOGY TIP

Sign off your office notes without re-reading or analyzing them.

Easier said than done, I know. So, start with something smaller, like email. Write an email to a friend and send it immediately without proofing it. This is a practice run. You will learn that 1) you didn't die. 2) no one criticized or judged you for that typo or grammatical error.

Then do it with notes. For an entire day force yourself to finish and sign off each note immediately, no proofreading, no editing. Ignore that itchy impulse to fix typos or formatting. By day's end, you will find all your notes completed and nothing left to take home. At first, it will feel strange and uncomfortable, but the more you practice doing this, the easier it will become.

DEALING WITH ATTENTION-DEFICIT ISSUES AND CHARTING

Computerized medical records can present a special challenge to someone who is prone to attention deficit disorder. For anyone with severe symptoms, it is best to seek professional help with a psychologist and to consider medication through a psychiatrist.

CLINICAL VIGNETTE:

A young Family Physician with previously diagnosed mild attention deficit disorder, not requiring medication, finds herself completely overwhelmed at work. She is falling behind in her charting despite seeing only 10-15 patients a day, and since she is transitioning from a base salary to an RVU-incentive salary, she is in danger of taking a financial loss unless she can increase her patient volume. She finds her electronic medical record particularly challenging because it requires many screen changes to look up and document information. She finds it difficult to focus on her patient and the computer at the same time, and often can't remember what she was looking for when she opens a different screen on the computer.

For milder ADHD symptoms, there are steps that can help your mind stay focused and organized when it comes to charting:

- It is especially important for those with ADHD to complete notes in real time
- Document the visit immediately after the patient encounter. Don't wait until later!
- Use the copy, paste, and edit technique for complex medical patients with multiple chronic health issues to stay on task
- Be diligent about getting out of the exam room as soon as possible.

Why? Because the longer you spend in the room, the more off-track you can become.

- Use your nursing staff to help you wrap up and transition out of the exam room.

PERFECTIONISM IN THE ELECTRONIC ERA

Many clinicians struggle with perfectionism. Being a perfectionist probably helped get us into medical school in the first place. And perfectionism is part of the conscientious and careful nature of the ideal physician. After all, who wants a doctor who isn't a bit of a perfectionist? *("I'll just check those lab results later, they're probably fine…")*

The challenge occurs when our perfectionism starts to take control of our lives. For example, we may begin to demand that every aspect of our efforts be perfect, when *"good enough"* will do. We may find ourselves struggling to complete our notes because they must be perfect before we sign them off. Or, we may set unrealistic *"all-or-nothing"* expectations for ourselves—*"if I can't get all these notes done today, then I am a failure and I should just give up."*

Change your thinking from fixed to growth mindset

The first step to dealing with perfectionism is to acknowledge that perfect is impossible. And, recognize the type of abnormal thinking involved in perfectionism. People who are perfectionists tend to have something that Carol Dweck termed as a "fixed" mindset, rather than a "growth" mindset.[xxii]

Fixed mindsets are all-or-nothing, black-or-white, and focused entirely on outcomes. So, if a perfectionist sees that they have three hundred clinic notes to complete, and it seems impossible to get a perfect result (completing all 300 in a short time frame), then she may just decide to give up and not even try.

Instead of having a fixed mindset, we need to work to changing our thinking towards the cultivation of a growth mindset. Growth mindsets change the focus from outcome results to an emphasis on effort and improvement. Instead of saying *"I'm a failure because I didn't finish all 300 charts,"* a growth mindset would say *"Wow! I got 20 charts done! I worked really hard. I just need to keep this up and I will get all my charts done."*

Get past image

Perfectionists struggle with self-image problems and tend to feel scrutinized and judged by others. This may extend to concerns over the appearance of clinic notes, which are often generated by electronic systems that include pages of useless information or unattractive formatting. Physicians fear that putting out an unprofessional appearing note will reflect negatively on their care. That then results in them spending excessive amounts of time trying to re-format and edit notes for a more desirable appearance.

Instead, change your thinking. Ask yourself, *"If I write this note and there is a grammatical error or typo, would another doctor really think less of me? Would a peer decide not to refer to me over something so minor?"*

While there may be a few physicians who would judge a colleague harshly for an ugly note, most of us don't care. We are simply reviewing notes looking for the information relevant to the care of our patients and ignoring the rest.

Perfectionists must train themselves to accept that for the most part, no one cares if their note is perfect. Our colleagues care only that the note is done, and that the essential information is somewhere in there. The rest is just, well, wasted time.

Dealing with fear and insecurity

Often perfectionism derives from a fear of repercussions, such as a malpractice lawsuit. And, it is understandable that physicians worry, as statistics show that most doctors will be sued—and some more than once—at some point during their career.[xxiii] While careful documentation can help in the event of a lawsuit, litigation may occur even if your notes are perfect. Even worse, when we focus so hard on *"not"* making a mistake, we often become distracted, and may actually increase our risk of a treatment error (discussed in more detail in chapter 16).

Another reason for procrastination may be less obvious—we may subconsciously fear our own success. Fear of success may seem counterintuitive, but it is a very real phenomenon.

First, fear of success stems from our fear of the unknown. Physicians often like to plan out every step of the future. We like to know what is going to happen and when. We don't like it when things don't go as expected, and we often fear change.

Being successful brings uncertainty. What changes will success bring to my life and will I be able to handle those changes? We fear the response from those jealous of our success as success can bring criticism and judgment. We may even lose friends and colleagues. Success sometimes brings loneliness as one separates themselves from the pack and is suddenly *"at the top."*

We also fear what may happen if we fail after being successful. What will others say? How will I recover?

And even more deeply, we may fear that once we finally do make the changes to succeed, we will feel guilty about not succeeding sooner, and dwell on potential wasted years of our lives.[xxiv]

The key to releasing fear of success is to *identify these feelings*. We need to analyze the concerns that hold us back, whether they are fear of negative repercussions, being criticized and judged, or of ultimately failing.

We also need to acknowledge that while there will be a few peers or colleagues who eagerly wait for us to fail to pounce, most of the people in our lives are either completely uninterested in us or hoping for our success. After all, if we succeed, then they can too!

And, if we do fail, we need to realize that forgiveness is built into our human nature. Think of all the badly behaving celebrities who turn their lives around and are forgiven and even celebrated by the public. We love to root for the underdog and nothing is better than a good comeback story.

FEELING GUILTY? STOP IT!

When we have hundreds of charts to finish, but we can't finish because of other things we believe must be attended to, we often feel powerful guilt.

Unfortunately, guilt is a horrible motivator. The more guilt we feel, the more likely is that we will continue to do the very thing we feel guilty about. So, stop feeling guilty and forgive yourself for being behind on your notes. It's not your fault that you don't have enough time and work in a terrible system.

On the other hand, you must take the responsibility to make positive changes, whether it's:

- documenting in a new way (more in the next section)
- cutting back on your schedule to allow more time to document adequately
- making a radical life change such as leaving your current job situation for something more manageable.

Regardless of what you decide, you *do* have a choice!

IMPROVE YOUR CHARTING, IMPROVE YOUR LIFE

CLINICAL VIGNETTE

A nurse midwife who has always loved her job and had top patient satisfaction ratings belongs to a practice that transitioned

> from paper charts to electronic health records. She finds herself increasingly behind in her charting and is now delinquent with hundreds of incomplete notes. She spends her evenings and weekends staring at her computer screen, feeling hopeless and depressed, no longer enjoys her job, and has even begun to have suicidal thoughts.

The best way to stay on top of charting: Get your notes done *in real time*. That means to document your notes during and after each patient encounter. Don't wait until the end of the day.

BUT THIS IS HARD!

It really is. It didn't used to be so hard. I hate to keep dragging us back to the paper and pen scenario, but the reality is writing by hand while listening to a person talk isn't that difficult. In fact, it is easy to jot a few notes while you nod your head empathetically and murmur *"hmm, tell me more about…"* You can scrawl all over a sheet of paper and keep most of your writing in line. You can also flip open a paper chart to check the date of the last tetanus shot or review the most recent labs, all while still giving eye contact to a patient. Not so with computer records.

First, it's very hard to type or click and talk to patients at the same time. If you try it, you may look down at the row of text you just typed and find that your fingers were on the wrong key and you just generated a row of gibberish. Sigh. Ok, backspace backspace backspace, try again. This time you pay more attention to your typing—don't want to repeat work again! So, you start to glance back and forth at the keyboard and less at your patient's face. Finally, you're just staring at the computer and not looking at your patient at all, and that's even worse!

THERE ARE SEVERAL SOLUTIONS TO THIS PROBLEM.

First, consider hiring a scribe.

USING A SCRIBE

Using scribes can improve physician productivity to the point where they pay for themselves. Most importantly, patients don't mind having a scribe in the exam room during their doctor visits.[xxv]

CLINICAL VIGNETTE

> I experimented with using a scribe when I worked at a busy RVU-based practice, using one of my medical assistants who was familiar with our EHR and my style of medical practice. The MA sat at the larger desktop computer, and her job was specifically to type/click data as I dictated it to her. I found that I needed to have a second laptop computer open to scroll through to check lab results, old notes, etc. in order to visualize the patient's history and keep myself on track.
>
> The biggest benefit to me was in dictating the assessment and plan, particularly when diagnostic codes needed to be looked up and entered, such as linking orders with diagnostic codes. The scribe would also print up lab orders, prescriptions, and patient information as I requested them. At the end of the patient encounter, the note was virtually complete, other than my quick review and sign-off.

A scribe can be a nonclinical staff member, a medical assistant, or a nurse. Several companies have cropped up that supply medical scribes, and there are even virtual scribes now.

It takes time to train a medical scribe. The scribe needs strong typing and computer skills and must be thoroughly trained in the electronic health system. Since each physician has a different style and documentation expectations, patience and detailed explanations will be critical.

The key to using scribes in an electronic system is to put them to work in the biggest sources of time drain for physicians. For most physicians, this is in computerized physician order entry (CPOE).

CPOE requires the doctor to search through a list of hundreds of tests to find and select the desired test code, and then to link that order with one of 68,000 ICD10 diagnostic codes ensuring that they pick the *"correct"* code—in other words, the one the insurer pays for. CPOE is an independent risk factor for physician burnout.[xxvi] Yet no proposals for reducing physician burnout has called for eliminating this stressor.

CPOE costs the system money because of the time it takes, and so one caveat is that if your company insists that physicians enter orders themselves and doesn't allow scribes to help, then the scribes will be less cost effective. This was shown by a hospital system that declined to allow scribes to enter orders into the computer system, and instead required physicians to continue to manually enter orders themselves. Because the scribes didn't end up saving the system money, the hospital canceled the program, even though physicians were happier and finishing documentation more quickly.[xxvii]

ROCK STAR TIP

If your company won't let your scribe enter orders, the scribe may no longer be as cost effective (but you will still be happier!).

DELEGATE DOCUMENTATION TO STAFF MEMBERS

Another option for delegating data entry is asking your nurse or medical assistant to enter information into the chart for you. This is particularly helpful when entering in historical information, such as the History of Present Illness (HPI) and past medical histories and medications. Some systems have kiosks or tablets that allow patients to enter information such as past medical history, family history, and review of systems.

Note that Medicare rules require a physician to obtain the History of Present Illness (HPI)[xxviii]—however, that doesn't mean that your nurse can't get preliminary information for you, which you can then explore in detail with the patient and edit in the note to make it "your own." The down side to this is that you will need adequate staff to be able to spend the time with your patients to obtain this information.

USE DICTATION

A third way to document in real time is to use dictation, and ideally to dictate in the presence of the patient. This ensures that you are entering accurate information and can be done using a conventional dictation service with a microphone or using a transcription computer program like Dragon.

DRAGON DICTATION TIPS

1. Get the very best microphone you can. An excellent microphone makes a tremendous difference in your dictation accuracy.
2. Train the Dragon. Dragon can learn, but it must be trained to your voice. Run the accuracy optimizer function frequently.
3. Create templates. Dragon can be very useful for creating templates of commonly used phrases, such as a generic treatment plan for viral infections and urinary tract infections. While it takes time to build these templates, you can get to a point where, with just a few words, you can create a complete note that can be edited and personalized for your patient.
4. Back up your work. Once you have created templates, back Dragon up or you may lose all your hard work in the event of a system crash.
5. Watch out for OCD/perfectionism. It is not uncommon to find that Dragon will randomly make errors like changing "he" to "she" or "will" to "we'll," no matter how well trained. Sometimes it types "C." when you meant "see," and it never knows if you wanted to

say "due" or "do." These types of grammatical errors can drive an OCD-type doctor crazy. You will have to use the perfectionism tips listed above to train yourself to ignore these mistakes and to avoid unnecessary time editing your notes.

6. Consider a disclaimer. Make a template to include at the end of all dictations: *"This note was generated using ___ EHR and dictated in part by ___ dictation program. Despite the best effort of the dictating physician, there may be grammatical or syntax errors."* Although it won't make any real difference, it might make you feel a little better.

USING MACROS/ QUICK-TEXTS

A great way to be more efficient in note-writing is to create your own macros or quick-texts. With a few key strokes, you can insert much more detailed text for a variety of commonly used phrases. Many electronic health systems allow users to create templates within the system, as does Dragon dictation. There are also text expanding programs which allow the development of more complex templates, which can be quickly edited and personalized. Several programs that get rave reviews from physicians are Breevy and TextExpander.

While it may take some time to create your own templates, the payoff can be huge. Why waste minutes of time typing the historical features of a cold or a urinary tract infection repeatedly when you can input the same information in within seconds? Although it may only take a minute or two to type each time, when you compound that time by a large volume of patient encounters, creating templates can save you a significant amount of time in the long run.

TYPING

Finally, if you choose to type (and some people really are great typists), practice using brief bullet points rather than writing complete sentences. Although this is usually easy to do when hand writing, it can be more of a challenge when typing. You must train yourself to be concise which requires more attention to the keyboard. And who really reads those extensive HPIs, anyway? By typing short phrases, you can more easily provide eye contact where it really needs to be directed—to the patient.

KEEP THE REVIEW OF SYSTEMS (ROS) AND PHYSICAL EXAM (PE) RELEVANT

Have you ever read an electronically generated physician note and rolled your eyes as you perused the review of systems and physical exam part? Pu-lease. It's so obvious that someone just clicked *"all"* in some engineered exam template, especially when the information contradicts itself or has an unreasonable amount of detail unnecessary to the chief complaint.

This type of documentation:

1. Looks bad, because obviously the examiner did not do everything the note indicates
2. Does nothing to protect you medicolegally
3. Makes it nearly impossible for another clinician to figure out if you found anything important on your exam.

If your system gives you no other choice than to select from a dropdown list of less-than-truthful elements, then put your foot down and tell your administrator NO. Because ultimately it is your license that is on the line, and an inaccuracy, even if computer generated by a bad system, can potentially be used to make you look like an uncaring or unethical physician in a legal case.

CLINICAL VIGNETTE

Dr. T was moonlighting at a facility that changed to a new EHR. The system wasn't intended for the type of medical practice it was being used for, and so the administration designed some work-arounds. One of these was a signature box that "verified" that physicians had performed a particular examination that wasn't a standard part of care in this type of practice. The system would not allow the chart to be closed until this box was

> clicked. Dr. T refused—"*I'm not going to acknowledge that I did something that I didn't do*," she insisted. The administrator was bewildered. "*But it's not a big deal—this isn't even a procedure that we do here.*" Ultimately, Dr. T had to leave the position because there was no alternative—the company had invested a huge sum in the system, and changing it wasn't an option. Getting Dr. T to compromise her medical license was even less of an option.

Keep your ROS and PE short and sweet by creating your own template of honest, commonly performed physical exam elements. Make sure that you only include what you really need to satisfy your medical decision making (MDM).

And, if you don't need the physical exam for your medical decision making, don't do it (sacrilege!). For example, a patient with depression may only require notation of general appearance, mood, and affect, and that's enough. Anything more is unnecessary and costs you time.

THE WHOLE POINT OF THE NOTE: DOCUMENTING MDM

From a billing perspective, the very best way to write our notes would be to start with MDM (or assessment and plan) and work our way backwards. Because every audit of coding accuracy is going to start at the same place: What is the level of medical decision making—straightforward, low, moderate, or high? Once that has been determined (and yes, there are a million rules on how this is calculated, because auditors are not physicians, after all), the auditor will then tally up your history and bullet points to see if they meet the threshold to warrant the code you submitted. It's crazy, but that's the current system that enables us to get paid by insurers.

So, the bottom line: Stop worrying so much about how much detail we put into our history and physical and focus more on the quality of our MDM. *Put your energy here when it comes to charting in real time.*

As you are talking with your patients, ask yourself if you are getting the information that you really need from your patient, with a focus on the medical care that you need to provide. It's ok to skip ahead to the assessment and to plan and start entering in diagnoses, medications, and lab orders as you talk with the patient.

It's also ok to ask the patient to pause in their history to focus on the MDM of a particular issue before moving on to their next issue so that you can get the information entered in real time. *"I want to hear about your cold, but first, let me make your lab orders to evaluate your diabetes and refill the diabetic medications."*

As soon as you have finished a patient encounter, enter your medical diagnoses and treatment plan. Do it while it is fresh in your mind, and remember to include a brief explanation of your thought process. This is the most important element in a malpractice suit—showing that you thought about more serious illnesses, why you ruled them out or how you plan to work them up. Be sure to include your recommendations for follow-up and instructions that you gave the patient. Templates and quick-texts can be especially useful when you give the same advice over and over, like warning a patient about what do to for recurrent or worsening symptoms.

Consider completing this part of your note in a separate area from the patient—sometimes the longer you sit in the exam room, the more questions and concerns the patient may bring up to you. Go from the exam room into your office or a quiet corner and complete your documentation prior to moving on to the next patient.

DOCUMENTING IN REAL TIME: DEALING WITH ANXIETY

A major reason that we often hesitate to complete our notes in real time is because we feel anxiety to get to the next patient. Maybe we are already running late and we know that we have many more patients to see. Or we could be getting pressure from administrators to generate more RVUs.

So, we decide to move on and do our notes later. Unfortunately, we are only deferring our anxiety by failing to do our notes in real time.

The best way to manage this is to *factor documentation time into your schedule*. If you are double, triple, and quadruple booked, you won't be able to get your notes done without spending hours at your computer after work. Accept that documenting is part of your job and a necessary component of every patient encounter. Notes don't just magically appear. They take time to complete. And that time must be calculated into your schedule.

PSYCHOLOGY TIP

Factor documentation time into your schedule.

JUST DO IT

Sometimes the only way to overcome your anxiety is to force yourself to sit down and do your note before moving on to the next patient. It's going to be painful, but it won't kill you. By the end of the day, you will have your notes complete and you can go home with nothing on your back, no homework to complete, and the rest of the evening at your disposal. Sounds good, doesn't it? Make it happen.

MAKE IT A HABIT

All habits must start somewhere. Start today by creating a challenge for yourself: *"Today, I'm going to get my charts done."* Do the best you can. Tomorrow, try again. If you don't get all your charts done, give yourself credit for what you did complete, and the progress that you've made. Be proud of your efforts and for trying to get your charts done. Every day that you succeed will make it easier to continue.

Practice using "if/then" statements. Rather than making vague statements like "I'm going to do better at getting my charts done," or "I need to get all my charts done today," say: "*If* I do not finish my charts by the end of the day, *then* I will stay late until they are done."

It may help to tell others what you are doing, such as your nurse or medical assistant. Or even to set up a challenge with one of your colleagues. Once you verbalize a goal, you are more likely to feel obligated and less likely to back out.

WHAT TO DO WHEN YOU ARE CATASTROPHICALLY BEHIND

CLINICAL VIGNETTE PART 2

> The nurse midwife, through heroic effort and with the help of an empathetic supervising physician, spent an entire weekend trudging through her backlog of charts, and completed her entire workload. She felt a tremendous sense of relief. She was able to stay on top of her charts for the next week or so, but by the next month, she found herself 30 charts behind. While she felt stressed, she also thought *"well, at least it's not 300 charts!"* Another month later, she was 50 charts behind. And within three months, her office manager was sending her regular emails and messages asking her about her charts again, and she began to feel aggrieved and anxious. The supervising doctor who helped her finish her charts was no longer as empathetic and the nurse was beginning to wonder if she was actually avoiding her.

Unfortunately, a person who is prone to getting catastrophically behind will continue to face this problem unless they take steps to change their day-to-day habits. They will also have to practice consistently enforcing the new way of charting, rather than procrastinating and leaving notes for later.

Before you can even begin to face a pile of late notes, you must make a plan for how you will face today's charts. Until you get control over how you are performing on a day-to-day basis, you will inevitably find yourself repeatedly playing catch up.

Think of a cross-country runner. A runner that starts late will sprint to catch up, but then will get tired, and find themselves lagging behind. Through a tremendous force of will, they may sprint again, trying to catch up, but then fall behind as fatigue kicks in. They will exhaust themselves trying to catch up and will never succeed.

So, start by learning how to complete notes in real time. Once you have a handle on getting today's charts completed by the end of the day, you can start to attack the older notes waiting to be completed.

How to play catch-up—setting realistic goals

Ask yourself how long it really takes you to complete a chart, and then use that information to set realistic goals. You may need to do a time awareness study to get a gauge on how long it really will take you (see Chapter 5). Once you know how long you really need, you can set your goals—if it takes you 10 minutes per chart, then give yourself a challenge to complete six charts in an hour.

If you expect yourself to complete 10 charts in an hour, but only have time to complete six, then you never experience a sense of success. At the end of the hour, you still have four charts left. As you look over those remaining charts, you feel a sense of failure, and this sucks away your motivation to continue.

Break up work into manageable chunks

Rather than thinking about the hundred charts you must complete, focus instead on completing ten charts. Once you've completed those charts, acknowledge your success! Feel a sense of gratification and acknowledge your accomplishment and effort.

While some companies will force delinquent employees to take a few days of vacation time to complete charts, this doesn't usually work. Instead, it's more realistic to spend a half hour or hour each day to focus on a small number of charts and complete them over a period of a few weeks. It's all about creating good habits, not cramming!

PSYCHOLOGY TIP

Don't take a day off work to play catch-up on charts. Instead, schedule 30-60 minutes per day until all your charts are complete.

Work where your brain functions the best

When possible, do your work where your brain works the best. Memory theory shows that we recall information better when we work in the setting or environment in which we learned it. Try to remember what you had for dinner last night. The first thing you will do is to think of where you were last night at dinner time—because your brain associates location with memory.

When you are working to catch up on charts, your brain must go back into the mode of where you were and what you were doing when you saw that patient. Most likely, this was in the clinic setting. So working from that location to catch up on your charts provides the best bet at recalling information quickly.

Clear away the clutter

Our brain works best with minimal clutter. This clutter can be external, like a messy desk or internal, with mental distractions such as email, social media or the presence of others. Work in a quiet setting. And avoid all distractions during the time that you set to do your charts. Set a timer for an hour. Congratulate yourself for your hard work. Then reward yourself with a break to go for a walk or meet a friend for coffee. But do not reward yourself with a computer break, which can be draining rather than refreshing. After you have had a break, sit down and focus on another manageable chunk of time without distractions.

Don't bring work home

Whenever possible, don't bring work home. It's often better to stay at work a little later than to take work home, as burnout occurs when you don't separate work and home. Working at home may impair your ability to sleep well and will cut into your relaxation time, which is necessary for quality of life.

PSYCHOLOGY TIP

Whenever possible, *don't bring work home.*

CAVEAT: In some cases, it may be necessary to take work home. Many parents of young children want to be home for dinner with the family and to get the kids to bed. In this case, do your charting in a separate part of the house, rather than in the family room or bedroom. And set a finite amount of time, like thirty minutes or an hour at most. Then give yourself a little buffer time between charting and going to sleep.

No more excuses

If you are often catastrophically behind, you may have a problem with simply not having enough time to do what you need to do. Ask yourself why—are you overextending yourself? Are you wasting time on nonessential tasks? Are you in a rut and mentally exhausted? Or are you simply working in a setting that has set you up for failure? Carefully analyze your situation. Ask yourself what personal changes you can make to escape from this mentally damaging pattern. Professional help may be warranted to help you get to the root cause and to take positive steps towards change.

PSYCHOLOGY TIP

Take the time to get help.

ROCK STAR ACTIVITY

Getting your notes done

At the end of the day, are your notes finished? If not, why?

____

____

What specific steps can you take to help you finish your notes?

____

____

List the barriers to not getting your notes done, and potential solutions:

SOLUTIONS

BARRIERS	SOLUTIONS

ROCK STAR ACTIVITY

Catching up on charts

First, make sure that your current notes are up-to-date. Next, make a schedule for completing delinquent charts and commit to getting your charts done during that time frame. If you have 100 charts to do, and it takes you 10 minutes to do each chart, schedule one hour per day and complete six charts. You will be done in just over two weeks!

Sample calendar: You decide the best time to do your notes is by spending 30 minutes each morning before work and 30 minutes at lunch, whenever possible. Looking at your calendar, you realize that some days you have other activities scheduled during those times, so you make the decision you will do your notes after work on those days. On the weekend, you plan to dedicate an hour each on Saturday and Sunday.

	Monday	Tuesday	Wednesday	Thursday	Friday	Saturday	Sunday
6AM	Chart 6-6:30	Chart 6-6:30	Meeting	Chart 6-6:30	Chart 6-6:30		
7AM							
8AM							
9AM							
10AM						**Chart 10-11**	**CHURCH**
11Am							

	Monday	Tuesday	Wednesday	Thursday	Friday	Saturday	Sunday
12PM	Chart 12-12:30	DENTIST	Chart 12-12:30	Chart 12-12:30	Chart 12-12:30		FOOTBALL
1PM						BARBECUE	↓
2PM						↓	↓
3PM						↓	↓
4PM						↓	↓
5PM						↓	↓
6PM						↓	Chart 6-7
7PM		Chart 7-7:30	Chart 7-7:30		DATENIGHT	↓	
8PM							
9PM							
10PM	BEDTIME	→	→	→	→	→	→

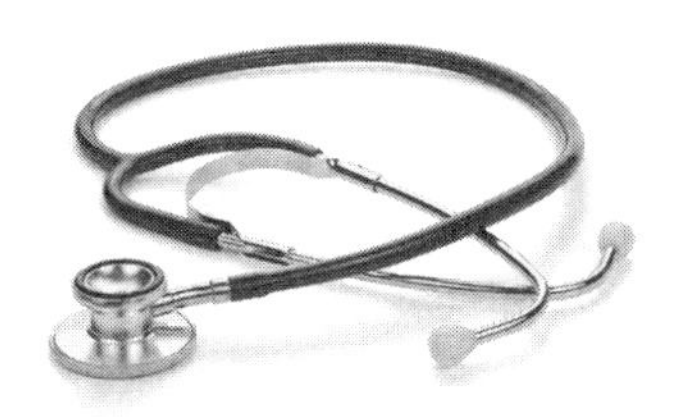

CHAPTER SEVEN

WORK-LIFE BALANCE: FIND YOUR INTRINSIC MOTIVATION

In Medscape's 2015 Physician survey, *"lack of professional fulfillment"* and feeling like a *"cog in the wheel"* ranked high among physicians' self-reported causes of burnout.[xxix]

As physicians have increasingly moved away from self-employment and into employed work, the locus of control has shifted away from an intrinsic motivation of solving problems and caring for patients and towards an extrinsic motivation of an outcome-based system. We now work either for a *"carrot:"* a reward of a paycheck for punching the clock and a bonus for a favorable patient-satisfaction survey, or a *"stick:"* such as a 5% pay cut for doctors whose patients don't quit smoking fast enough, and a fine for the doc who fails her Medicare audit.

Unfortunately, carrots and sticks are horrible motivators. That's why schemes like pay-for-performance are destined to fail. Human beings just aren't wired that way. Once we achieve the promised reward, our motivation to continue declines and our intrinsic drive shrinks.[xxx] We resent those sticks, so we sometimes resort to scheming and deviousness to avoid punishment.

What works much better is intrinsic motivation, something that doctors have in spades, at least when we are starting out. It's what we wrote about in our personal essays to get into medical school—all about our hopes and dreams, how we were going to save the world, and help our fellow man. You remember, before your hopes and dreams were crushed under a mountain of bureaucracy and paperwork.

But, wait! Our intrinsic motivation still lives. It's just pushed down a bit deeper. So we may have to dig down to retrieve it. We must find what interests us, what gives us meaning and purpose. We need a personal goal, something that we can invest in, and that gives us a reason to work other than a paycheck.

PSYCHOLOGY RULE #4

Find your intrinsic motivation.

According to the Mayo Clinic, spending 20% of your work time on that intrinsic motivator (or, aspect of work that you find the most meaningful) has a powerful effect on reducing burnout.[xxxi] If you are passionate about working with the underserved, spend a day a week in a rural clinic or homeless shelter. If you love to write, do some part-time medical blogging—just find your 20%!

PSYCHOLOGY TIP

Find your passion and spend 20% of your work time on it.

We must also learn to refocus our thinking from an outcome-based mindset to a growth-based mindset. This means acknowledging not only our accomplishments but also our efforts. Look at how far you have come from that pre-med student who wrote that incredibly naïve personal statement. Recognize your growth and improvement and take pride in your hard work. The happiest people use themselves as a yardstick for internal evaluation.

Now create a vision of growth for yourself. Where do you want to be in a year? In five years? In ten? Ask why you are doing what you are doing. Ask what you need to feel satisfied. What made you want to be a doctor in the first place? It might be the problem-solving element, hearing patient stories or being intellectually challenged. Determine how you can incorporate and emphasize those elements into your practice every day, and not just 20% of the time.

Once you find more intrinsic motivation for your work day, it's time to figure out the next step—how to get out of the office and create a life outside of work. Ask yourself: *Where do you want to be, and what do you need to do to get there?*

ROCK STAR ACTIVITY

Intrinsic motivators and your "20%"

What are your intrinsic motivators? ______________________

____

____

____

____

What is your 20%? ______________________________

____

____

____

____

What is your first step to instituting a plan? ____________

____

____

____

____

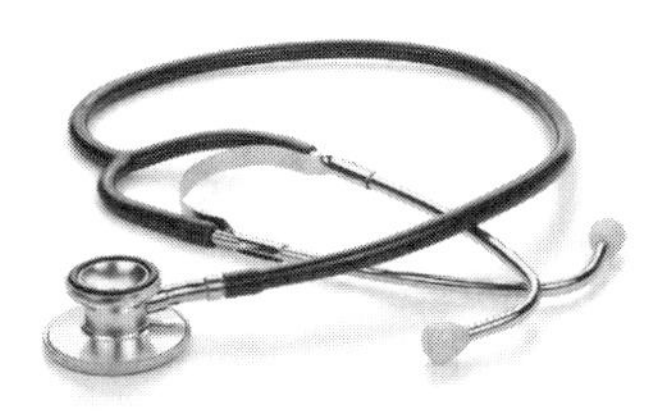

CHAPTER EIGHT

USE PSYCHOLOGY TO FIND WORK-LIFE BALANCE—FINDING HAPPINESS OUTSIDE THE OFFICE

Physicians struggle more with work-life balance than other US workers, in large part due to an increased number of work hours. In fact, about 50% of US physicians work more than 60 hours per week, compared with under 10% for other professionals.[xxxii]

However, our challenge with work-life balance stems from more than mere work hours: It also has much to do with the psychology of the physician persona, including our issues with martyrdom, perfectionism, insecurity, and social isolation.

Martyrdom in medicine

Medical training requires intense self-sacrifice and delayed gratification. And, it can lead to an intense sense of indispensability. Our importance in the hospital setting fuels our ego and satisfies our core human need to be appreciated, wanted, and *"in demand"* from others. We feel proud of our abilities and this boosts our confidence.

The satisfaction that we gain from being needed in our physician role can become so strong that it overpowers other elements in our lives. Often, we may start to perceive our work as the most important aspect of our being. As work becomes more and more important, we may find ourselves sacrificing relationships with family and friends, our own hobbies and interests, and even our own health.

Perfectionism and insecurity

Physicians tend to be both highly perfectionistic and incredibly insecure. We constantly worry about whether we are good enough, and whether we will make a mistake. When we face stress in our lives, we sometimes respond by turning towards the things we are good at. For many physicians, that means work. Work also provides a sense of security that we crave, especially as many physicians dread change.

When we are stressed, we often latch onto what we do well and are good at. For example, if a physician struggles in business, he may find himself overscheduling clinical hours because this is an area in which he excels, and in which he feels more confident and comfortable.

Social isolation

Lee Lipsenthal MD points out that many physicians become *"social isolates."*[xxxiii] He attributes this tendency to an introspective personality type, combined with years of intense study and work when our peers are much more focused on relationships and social activities. Physicians often withdraw from social situations and instead focus on work, particularly when feeling overloaded. This social isolation makes it even more difficult for us to develop a life outside of work hours.

USE PSYCHOLOGY TO FIND WORK-LIFE BALANCE

To achieve work-life balance, physicians first must develop self-awareness into why they spend so many hours at work. This is hard, because it requires you to acknowledge your faults and weaknesses, rather than focusing on your strengths. You must identify areas of avoidance and ask yourself why you shy away from certain activities. Finally, you must pay attention to your actions and how others respond to you.

If you find yourself staying late at work all the time, ask yourself why. Are you procrastinating going home? Maybe you have no hobbies. Maybe you don't do anything fun anymore. Or maybe you don't feel like dealing with your family. If so, acknowledge the reasons and start working on them. Quit avoiding the real issue by hiding from it at work.

PSYCHOLOGY TIP

If you are a workaholic, ask yourself *why*. What are the possible reasons behind your decision to work all the time?

RELATIONSHIPS

Overwork can lead to relationship problems, especially if one partner uses work as an excuse to avoid responsibilities at home or nurturing family bonds. Remember that every relationship in which an individual engages must satisfy core needs. Even the most altruistic-seeming relationship satisfies needs. If a physician gets their emotional needs satisfied through our profession or occupation, we may ignore other relationships, even in our own family.

Avoid alienating your partner

One of the challenges that physicians face is alienating our partners by shutting them out of our lives. Doctors tend to respond to workplace stress by trying to separate completely from work when at home. So, when our spouse asks us about our workday, we may shut them off because we don't want to think or talk about work once we are home.

Unfortunately, this attempt at complete separation causes a dual identity inside the physician, with both sides struggling for dominance. The clinician, sometimes with the best intention, may end up coming off as condescending and cold, not wanting to share our life with our partners. This creates a barrier which can lead to our partner not sharing their lives with us and an inability to grow as a couple.

Share your feelings

Sometimes we choose not to share the negatives in our life, such as financial stress, because we don't want to burden our partners. This noble intention can cause a relationship rift because it doesn't allow others in our life to offer support. Ultimately, that leads to our own isolation. We start to feel inadequately supported and resentful towards our partners. And they, in turn, feel criticized and rejected.

One of the reasons we don't always share our situation with our partners is the sense that *"they won't understand what I'm going through,"* especially if they are non-medical. However, we don't need to get into details or medical procedures to share the emotions that we are feeling. For example, if we lose a patient, we don't have to describe the entire medical scenario. We can simply say *"I'm feeling very sad and guilty about a patient's death."* We need to share our feelings so that our partners can be our support and trust them to be supportive, which they can't do if we don't let them.

Conversely, we also need to share the good as well as the bad. *"One of my patients wrote a nice review about me on our website—it made me feel really good."* By sharing positives with those close to us, we can get their validation rather than seeking it from others in less healthy ways.

Show an interest

One of the best ways to improve a relationship is to simply show an interest in our partners' lives. Just because our partner isn't a physician or works at home doesn't mean that they don't put just as much effort and determination into what they do. Try to understand how their day has gone. And spend some time talking about what interests them.

Take an active role in your partner's social life

Get to know more about your partner's friends and family. Doctors often know more about their secretary and nurse's kids than they do about their own spouse or kids. This is partly because we spend more time at work than we do at home. Get to know more about your partner to feel more connected and to improve your relationship.

Do stuff together

Plan activities together that aren't tied to work. Physicians often drag their spouses to networking events and physician meetings. But this doesn't really count as *"quality time"* for the partners. Find something fun that you can both enjoy. Make sure that not every vacation is a business trip or CME activity.

Acknowledge that your spouse needs time off too

Physicians work hard and we come home tired. It's easy to get resentful if we are asked to watch the kids or do housework as soon as we walk in the door. But we must realize that our spouse has been working hard all day too. So, they also need a break in addition to adult interaction.

Make an agreement that when you come home, you take twenty or thirty minutes to decompress and then take over with kid duty or help with dinner. Or, maybe you need to consider getting some household help so that both of you can get time off together. After all, that's what partnership is about.

RELATIONSHIPS AND WOMEN PHYSICIANS

Work-life balance can be particularly challenging for women who need to juggle their professional role with their roles as spouse and mother. This role strain creates powerful internal conflict with feelings of guilt about being inadequate at work and at home.

The struggle is real: Women do take on a much greater burden of household and child care compared to their male colleagues. That's partially because men physicians are more likely to have a stay-at-home spouse who handles home chores.[xxxiv] [xxxv]

Women doctors report a sense of obligation to spend more time at home and to make greater adjustments to their work schedule in order to manage household tasks than their male counterparts.[xxxvi] Women are more likely to make a career change to accommodate their spouse's career or child raising responsibilities.[xxxvii]

DEFINE ROLES AND RESPONSIBILITIES

Role conflict is the juggling act of balancing our various roles – physician, spouse, parent, housekeeper, short order cook, etc. The clearer the lines between roles and the less we must sacrifice one role for the other, the happier we are. Communication between women and their partners is essential to minimize role strain. Specifically defining roles and responsibilities—who does what around the house—is helpful in reducing burnout in women, especially before children come into the picture.[xxxviii]

Ask for help and accept help from your partner

Sometimes women suffer from a martyrdom complex—that only they can do the job or do the job right. To prevent burnout, women must ask for help and allow their partners to carry out responsibilities without micromanaging or getting frustrated that tasks aren't accomplished exactly the way that they would have done it.

CLINICAL VIGNETTE

Dr. N, a busy Family Physician, was exhausted working full time and managing most of the child raising duties for her son. For the first eight years of his life, she felt as if her entire weekends were taken up with kid activities like sports practice, piano lessons, and play dates, while her internal medicine physician husband spent his weekends on the couch watching football. After their divorce and custody agreement, dad started taking their son every other weekend and for a month during the summer. Although it took some getting used to for Dr. N to trust that her son would be cared for, eventually Dr. N began to feel she had a little bit of her own life back. *"I went on my first real vacation in years,"* she said. *"My stress level is better, and I'm happier at work now that I have some weekends free to relax a little."*

Use financial resources

Women should use their financial resources to get help with managing role strain. You can't do it all yourself. So, whenever possible, get help—for child care, house cleaning services or ordering out meals to avoid cooking. Don't feel guilty. Think of it as a value proposition. Physician time is best compensated when working as a physician. Then, let yourself relax and spend time with your family. That will make you more effective during your work hours.

Get a prenup

Women physicians also have higher rates of divorce then men with the chance of divorce increasing with their number of work hours.[xxxix] While the strain of separation and a divorce puts women at high risk for burnout, sometimes women physicians stay in a miserable marriage because of the financial penalties that divorce incurs. Getting a prenup won't prevent all the pain of a divorce, but it certainly makes it much easier. A prenup can:

- help you avoid paying alimony in many states
- protect your medical practice
- keep you from having to pay your spouse's debts
- lower attorney fees
- speed divorce proceedings, which is really important when you just want to move on with your life.

CLINICAL VIGNETTE

Dr. M, a midlife OBGYN discovered that her husband of 20 years and stay-at-home dad, was having an affair. *"You can divorce me,"* he said when she confronted him, *"but according to my lawyer, you're going to have to pay me alimony to 'keep me in the lifestyle to which I've been accustomed.'"* Dr. M was horrified to find that in her state, this was true. Adultery had no bearing on alimony payments. Not only that, but divorce would require a 50:50 split of everything she owned, including the family home and retirement fund that she had been contributing to for her entire career. She decided that staying in the marriage and living in separate bedrooms was less financially ruinous than divorcing.

Quit being so hard on yourself!

Women doctors must learn to lower our own self-expectations. This might be the toughest of them all. But it is vital to acknowledge that absolutely no one can *"do it all."* Talking with fellow women physicians can be helpful to realize that you are not alone, and finding a good psychologist can also help. Learn how to let go of the guilt of not being the perfect doctor, wife, and mother. Also learn how to prioritize your time, practice saying *'no'* before you feel overwhelmed, and take care of yourself so that you can take care of others.

PARENTING AND WORK-LIFE BALANCE

Raising children can be incredibly challenging, especially as a physician tries to balance a demanding work schedule with the needs of his or her children. For women, being a mom is so stressful that women physicians report the best mental health when the kids turn 19—or in other words, leave home![xl]

The most important factors affecting physician satisfaction with child raising are the amount of role conflict that we face and whether we have a supportive spouse.

When it comes to balancing family and work, one technique that can help is to ask yourself: *"Why am I working?"* If the answer is to provide financially for the family, ask yourself if you are working more than you need to achieve that goal. Can you reduce your work load so that you can have more time at home?

Fathers especially need to prioritize time with children. Providing financially is not enough and is not even the most important role of a father. When dads are supportive and take on more childrearing responsibilities, moms are happier and have less burnout. But even more importantly, a wealth of data shows that the more involved fathers are in the day-to-day lives of their children, the more successful their children will be in the future.[xli] Just getting involved in everyday activities, such as eating dinner together and playing together makes a difference.

Play with your kids

For young children, just ten minutes of uninterrupted one-on-one play with each child, done by each parent, provides tremendous psychological benefits. Let your kid pick what they want to do and just go along with it. Get on the floor or sit at the table, and act like a sports commentator, narrating what they are doing and copying their actions. *"I see you are putting the blue Legos together; I'm going to do that too!"* In this activity, the parent should not ask questions or give directions. Your job is to follow the child's lead and simply participate as you narrate the activity.

CLINICAL VIGNETTE

Dr. C, a physician mom of three who worked part-time was called into school for behavioral problems with her six-year old. She took him to a psychologist who asked Dr. C if she ever played with him. *"Well, we read together every night,"* she answered. *"And I take him to the park every day and he plays on the playground." "But do you actually get down on the ground with him and play the kind of games that he wants to play?"* the therapist asked. Dr. C was open to trying. That night, she invited her son up into the playroom, leaving the other two kids with dad. *"What would you like to play?"* Her son was taken aback at first but was quick to warm to the idea. Soon, they were racing matchbox cars on the floor and building castles out of tinker toys. *"It was actually pretty fun,"* said Dr. C, *"but more importantly, after a few weeks, I could see behavioral improvements in my son. The school stopped calling me, and he seems much happier. I look forward to coming home to see the kids."*

Show interest in your children's lives

How many doctors do you think only went to medical school because it's something that their parents pressured them into doing? Probably more than a few. Perhaps this relates to the high burnout levels that physicians face.

Don't try to force your interests on your kids. Conversely, just because your interests don't overlap doesn't mean that you shouldn't take an active role in what your kids enjoy. Be open-minded about your children's interests. Doctors are notoriously bad at this, but practice will strengthen your relationship with your children.

CLINICAL VIGNETTE

Dr. J loved golf and dreamed of bringing a future son or daughter to the golf course with him. *"It's embarrassing, but I actually had a little fantasy about what it would be like."* His daughter had different plans. Despite his best efforts (private golf lessons, personalized clubs), she detested the sport. *"I kept trying and trying to get her to like it, and it would end up in screaming fights. It was really disappointing to me. I had to accept that my dream was not going to come true and try to find things to do together that she enjoyed."*

GET A LIFE

PSYCHOLOGY RULE #5

Develop and maintain personal hobbies outside of medicine.

Enjoying hobbies and activities outside of medicine is one of the best ways to improve quality of life and mental health. Creative outlets like writing, knitting and crochet, cooking new recipes, painting, drawing, sketching, and musical performance have been found to improve emotional wellbeing and creativity.[xlii] These creative activities are wonderful for physicians who spend all day thinking analytically and can benefit from a mental break.

Hobbies provide all sorts of benefits—they stimulate our brain to learn something new, expand our social connections, and just make us all-around more interesting.

If you think that you don't have time for a hobby, think again. Scheduling time for hobbies forces us to be more efficient and productive during our available time so that we waste less time on passive and less useful activities like television and scrolling through Facebook.

So, get beyond networking and medical meetings and find something fun to do. What did you enjoy before medical school? When was the last time you read for pleasure? What do you feel you are missing out on or what have you always wanted to do?

If you want to spend more time outdoors, plant a garden or join a birdwatching group. To stimulate your brain, learn a language or musical instrument. For a healthy creative outlet, take a dancing lesson. Or, if you just want to get into a pleasant mental flow, work on a jigsaw puzzle or build a model airplane. Get online to see what events are going on in the community. If you're feeling particularly adventurous, check out a website like Groupon or Meetup and see what deals or groups you can find—maybe you will bungee jump for the first time or take a pole dancing class—who knows?

Do something just because you can

It can be very therapeutic to do something impulsive or silly—like jumping into a photo booth at the mall and taking goofy pictures with your spouse or laying on the ground and finding images in the clouds. Don't get so caught up in the everyday and practical.

Maintain ties with friends and family

It seems challenging to stay connected when we are so busy and tired but maintaining ties with our friends and family provides a great deal of emotional support. The key is to reach out as soon as you think about that person—make the time now for a quick phone call or a hello email or even a text to schedule a time to talk. Sometimes the longer it's been since we've connected, the harder it is to make that phone call. But, you can rekindle real friendships even after time lapses, so don't put it off any longer.

PSYCHOLOGY TIP

The moment a friend or family member pops into your mind, take the opportunity to reach out. If the timing isn't right for a phone call, at least send a text or email.

Take a break

Get season tickets to the local sports team or theater. Schedule yourself a massage or facial once a month. Have poker night with the boys on Fridays. Plan a date night with your spouse on Saturdays. Whatever you choose to do, schedule yourself time for fun and recreation. Mark it in your calendar so that it's set in stone—cell phones off and no work on date night!

Schedule time off during the work week

Schedule a half day or even a full day off from work every week to take care of your own needs. Everyone inevitably needs some time off during those typical 9-5 office hours for medical appointments, dentist visits, post office runs, and banking. Use this time to take care of yourself.

Schedule breaks at work

It's tough to be compassionate with patients or efficient with charting when you're hungry, thirsty or deferring bodily necessities. Doctors are not superheroes. We are human beings, and we need to eat, and drink, and use the bathroom just like everyone else. It's ridiculous to even need to state this. Yet what physician schedule factors in breaks for our basic human needs?

Take five or ten minutes a few times a day to have a snack or a drink, stretch your legs or do some breathing exercises. Close your office door, walk down to the break room, or go outside for a breath of fresh air. Build this time into your schedule or set an alarm to trigger you to take a short break. Breaks are necessary, and they make us more productive.[xliii]

Look for opportunities for breaks. If you are at the hospital making rounds and a nurse is in the room with a patient, rather than interrupting, take the opportunity to sit in a quiet area for five minutes. Get some alone time in the stairwell by taking the stairs rather than the elevator for a moment of peace. Or if you pass by a particularly pleasant looking garden, stop to smell the roses.

Take sick days when you need them

Physicians are notorious for dragging ourselves into work, even when we are deathly ill. It probably starts during our medical school or residency days—we can't possibly let our teammates down, so we drag ourselves into the hospital. It can even become a perverse source of bragging rights: *"You came in to work with a 103-degree fever? Well, one time I had to hook myself up to IV fluids, give myself a liter of saline, and then go back down to the ER to admit patients."*

Sociologists have a name for this type of behavior: *presenteeism*. And, it ain't good. Economists say that coming in to work sick actually costs the system money by decreasing our productivity and worsening our mental health.[xliv] Working while you are sick doesn't do anyone any good. Worse, it can take an overall toll on your physical and emotional well-being. If you are sick, take the day off, for everyone's sake.

Vacation

Taking regular vacations protects against the long-term health effects of chronic work stress, with certain caveats.[xlv] First, vacation time must allow a physician to mentally detach completely from work. That means no work-related phone calls, emails, texts or conference calls. Secondly, studies show that the benefit of vacation is negated by high levels of workload upon returning from vacation. So, ensure adequate coverage from a colleague and plan for a day or two just to deal with paperwork before getting back to *"regular"* work.

PSYCHOLOGY TIP

The best vacation for beating burnout involves getting *far away* from work and avoiding work responsibilities completely! CME trips and business meetings don't count.

Other variables to a successful vacation include planning ahead, creating social connections on your trip, going far away from work, and feeling safe.[xlvi] Many physicians enjoy joining organized tour groups, which take care of the planning for you, provide for safety within the group, and introduce you to new friends.

CONSIDER WORKING FEWER HOURS

When I talk about physician burnout to medical societies, there is almost always a physician who raises his or her hand at the end of the lecture and suggests doctors should consider working fewer hours. It's usually a doctor approaching retirement age who says, *"I finally learned to just work less and accept a lower paycheck to be happier."* Indeed, evidence has shown that reducing work hours may help some physicians to reduce burnout. [xlvii]

If you are feeling overwhelmed with work, cutting your schedule back may be a viable solution. Maybe you can simply carve out a half day or a day per week of administrative time to get your charting and paperwork done. Or, perhaps you feel you need a drastic reduction in work hours to part-time status to improve your quality of life.

First, meet with your financial advisor and make a financial plan. Find out exactly what level of earning you need to meet your expenses and plan for your future. Can you survive on a lower income? Or, can you cut your spending to compensate? Figure out exactly how much you must work to earn the income you need. If you are working more hours than you need to, consider cutting back to spend more time on yourself and your family.

If you do cut back to part time, or even decide to retire, consider how you will spend the extra time. Be sure to replace that time with something meaningful. Doctors who retire and find themselves twiddling their thumbs often become more depressed.

The key to easing out of work is replacing work hours with alternate activities that give your life value and meaning. This can be spending time with family or friends, working in the community, taking classes, doing something creative, traveling, teaching or any activity that piques your interest. This new free time is your time!

But, before we can get the chance to stop working so much and start living the life that we want to live, we must figure out how to bow out of the activities that no longer interest us. That can be difficult for physicians, who often have a difficult time saying *'no.'*

ROCK STAR ACTIVITY

Find a hobby outside of medicine

List out five things you have always wanted to do, but have "never had the time," or have had some excuse not to do (example: learn to play the piano, go for walks on the beach).

1.____

2.____

3.____

4.____

5.____

Now pick one of these hobbies and schedule time to commit to doing it. Don't just squeeze it into your schedule!

ROCK STAR ACTIVITY

Know your NNW

What is your "NNW?"—***number needed to work.*** In other words, how many hours do you need to work in a week to cover your expenses and desired quality of life?

Don't just guess. Schedule an appointment with an expert, like a financial advisor who works with physicians, to get the hard facts. Use this information to decide if you can cut back your work hours or consider making a change to an alternate career path (see chapter 19).

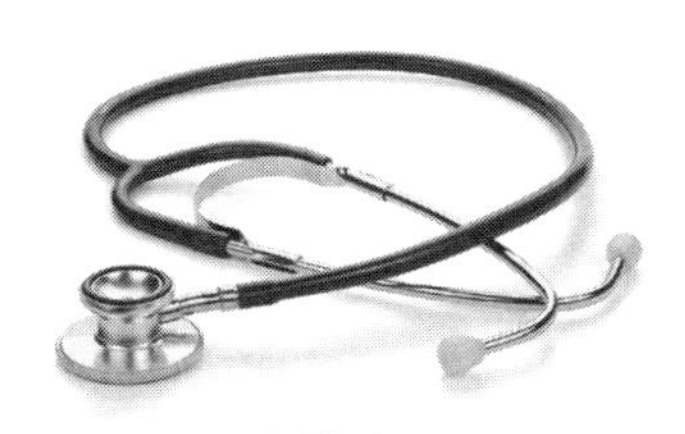

CHAPTER NINE

HOW TO SAY 'NO' AND WHEN TO SAY 'YES'

Physicians who struggle with work-life balance often find that they overcommit because they have difficulty saying no. Inability to say *'no'* is a tremendous cause of stress and burnout for physicians. We must learn to find and set boundaries to reduce burnout and improve mental health.

PSYCHOLOGY RULE #6

Boundaries are our friend.

CLINICAL VIGNETTE

Dr. A was approached by the administration of her large group and invited to participate on a committee to improve the Electronic Health Record. She agreed, flattered to have been considered and feeling a sense of responsibility to her colleagues to make their lives easier. Dr. A attended monthly meetings and provided recommendations for changes to make the system more efficient, which were promised to be investigated by the IT team. The meetings occurred after-hours and were uncompensated, which Dr. A found annoying, but she decided that the sacrifice would be worthwhile if positive changes resulted from her input. Unfortunately, little real change occurred, and a year later an announcement was made at a staff meeting that the company would be changing to a completely different electronic health record. Dr. A found herself filled with anger—all the meetings and time wasted, for nothing. She sat through the rest of the meeting in a blind rage and heard nothing else during the meeting. She was so frustrated and angry that she could barely get through her clinic day, and even found it hard to be civil to her patients and staff.

When we don't know how to say no (or when we say yes for the wrong reasons), we often end up resentful and angry, which takes a toll on our psyche. There are a multitude of psychological reasons that keep us from just saying 'no,' even when we are overworked and overextended. The common denominator is often fear.

Fear of not making others happy

Physicians are often notorious people-pleasers and we have anxiety about not making someone happy or satisfied. This may stem from childhood associations and desire to please our parents who may have had high expectations of us. It can also come from societal pressure of *"the customer is always right,"* like patient satisfaction surveys and doctor review sites.

Fear of losing job or status

We often say *'yes'* to undesirable requests from our employers because we fear that if we refuse, we may get fired or lose our status at work. Or, we take on extra shifts or work because we fear not having enough money. Unfortunately, we say yes so often that when we finally hit our limit, we become angry and blow up. We then find ourselves labeled as a *"disruptive"* physician, which ends up leading to trouble or even job loss.

Fear of missing out

Another reason we hesitate to say no is that we fear missing out or because we think that we are the only person who can do the job right. So, when we are asked to be involved in activities that don't really interest us, we sometimes say yes because we worry: *"If I say no today, I'll never be asked again, and I may miss out on a future opportunity."* Alternately, we may fear that someone else who we don't trust will take the role.

Fear of being inadequate or incapable

On a deeper level, saying no may be difficult because we associate it with a lack of knowledge. By saying no, we subconsciously fear that we are presenting ourselves as being incapable. *"I should be able to say yes—if not, it means I'm weak,"* or not smart enough or not good enough.

Fear of conflict

A major reason that physicians won't say 'no' is to avoid conflict. This may relate to our people pleasing tendencies or because we dread confrontation. We may fear that someone will be upset with us or that we will let them down. We may find it easier in the moment simply to agree to whatever demand is asked. Unfortunately, this leaves us with the angst of feeling stuck doing something we don't really want to do, and then we feel internal anger and frustration.

OVERCOMING FEAR AND LEARNING TO SAY "NO"

The first step to taking back control of your decisions is to ask yourself: What makes you afraid of saying no? Examine your anxieties and fears.

Determine if they are realistic or if you are wandering into catastrophic thinking.

CLINICAL VIGNETTE

A physician grew up in poverty, and even though she has a good income and is on track with savings and retirement, she finds herself unable to say *'no'* to every extra shift that she is offered on weekends. Any time she contemplates saying *'no,'* she suddenly gets anxious that in the future something bad might happen—she might lose her job or get sick—and she will end up poor like she was in her childhood, so she had better take every opportunity she can *"just in case."* However, she is becoming exhausted with working seven days a week and it's taking a toll on her relationships and free time.

Catastrophic thinking compounds the fear of saying 'no.' For example: "*If I don't agree to serve on this committee, I will get fired from my job, I won't be able to find a new job, I'll lose my home, etc.*" Or *"If I don't cover the shift for Dr. Jones, he will be annoyed with me and might tell others not to send me referrals."*

Practice feeling OK when you say no

Fortunately, we can learn to change our thinking through mindful practice. Instead of thinking catastrophically, practice thinking more realistically and more positively about the result of you saying *'no.'* For example, instead of imagining Dr. Jones being angry at you when you say that you can't cover his shift, visualize Dr. Jones saying with a smile, *"No problem, I'll check with someone else."* Instead of feeling guilty about saying no, practice deliberately feeling calm and comfortable with your decision and the outcome. Imagine everything going back to normal and all is well.

Don't overexplain

This is going to sound crazy to some, but it's ok to say no just because you want to—*you don't need a reason*. On top of that, here's something even more radical: it's not necessary to explain why you are saying no. In fact, it can be detrimental to explain your rationale because this gives the other person room to manipulate us, since they get the feeling that we can be talked into doing what they want us to do. Resist the temptation to explain, justify, or conciliate. Just say no.

PSYCHOLOGY RULE #7:

'No' is a complete sentence.

Understand your motivations

If you are going to say no (or yes!), know why. It might be because you just don't feel like doing it, or there could be a more complex rationale. You don't have to explain it to anyone, but it helps to think about your own motivations. Why am I agreeing to this activity? What value does it bring me? Does it align with my future goals?

Also consider the way that those around you influence your decisions. For example, if an administrator is asking you to do something in front of your peers, you may feel pressured to say yes. Or maybe you just came out of a meeting where your group was lectured about getting more involved with company activities—this may affect your decision when the boss comes walking down the hall to ask you to join the latest corporate committee.

Missing out is not the end of the world

We often agree to every offer because we fear if we say no, we will stop being asked. Sometimes this is true. However, it's not necessarily a bad thing. It's far better to plan to seek out opportunities that interest you, rather than getting sucked into more and more low value activities that come with saying 'yes' to every invitation.

PSYCHOLOGY TIP

Instead of saying yes to low value activities, plan to seek out opportunities that interest you.

Stop playing the martyr

I'm sorry to be the one to tell you this, but you are not indispensable. When you are long gone, someone else will chair that committee and head up that task force. We must fight the anxiety that stems from thinking that we are the "only" person who can do the job (or do the job right), which compels us to take on every offer and opportunity that presents itself until we are so burned out that we can't manage our regular responsibilities or take care of ourselves.

Bite the bullet and 'just say no'

Fear of confrontation and conflict is a huge problem for many of us. We may dread conflict so much that we will agree to something quickly only to spend hours scheming on ways to get out of doing it, making ourselves miserable in the process. The good news is that saying 'no' gets easier the more you practice doing it. Practice saying 'no' mentally, going through the exercise of positive thinking—as you say 'no,' you feel relaxed, you don't feel guilty, you are not overexplaining, and the person you say no to takes it well. Now do it for real.

USE PSYCHOLOGY LIKE A BOSS

It's hard to say no to a person in a position of power over you. Here are some psychology tips to make it easier.

Say 'no' by saying 'yes'

Instead of saying no, say yes in exchange for something that you want. There are two benefits to this technique. First, it places the control in your hands by putting pressure on the person asking for the favor to do something for you. Second, and more importantly, the person asking for the favor often won't want to make the trade and may just decide to rescind the request.

For example, an administrator asks you to serve on a committee that meets at 6 pm. You respond: *"I would love to! I'll just need you to block my schedule at 3 pm so I can make it on time."* This puts the onus on the administrator now to determine if blocking your schedule is something she is authorized to do or if it's more trouble than it's worth—and she may just find some other sucker, I mean, doctor, to ask.

This technique works great in the household too. *"Can you pick up the kids from school?" "Absolutely! I was just starting the laundry—if you can take it over, I'll run over and get the kids."* Request rescinded.

PSYCHOLOGY TIP

Say no by saying yes: offer to make a trade for something that you want or need.

Offer a little resistance

When someone is asking you for a favor or request, they usually want an easy yes response without a ton of questions. Offering a little resistance, like asking for more information to think about before you decide, may motivate the asker to move on to someone else.

Asking questions can also buy you time to come up with good reasons why you wouldn't necessarily be the right person for a particular job. Instead of immediately agreeing to sit on a committee, for example, have the asker give you more details about the committee and what the group is looking for in members. As you listen to the details, see if there is some reason why you wouldn't be a good fit.

Know the tricks

Every MBA includes plenty of courses on negotiation, so it makes sense that administrators have the edge over physicians in the boardroom. Learning some of the tricks of negotiation can help. First, avoid meeting your boss in their office. Instead, if they request a meeting, ask them to come to your office, where you will feel more in control. Make sure that they sit down when you meet.

Second, avoid agreeing to any requests when you are too busy or distracted to make a good decision. For example, administrators are infamous for showing up unannounced at your office while you are in the middle of a busy clinic day. While greeting them graciously is always wise, avoid agreeing to any requests or having any meetings right at that moment. Instead, ask them to schedule a time when you are free to think without distractions, saying *"It sounds like this is important. I don't have time right now to give it the attention it needs."*

Know that administrators will sometimes ask for favors and pressure you to answer without providing you adequate information. This works in their favor, as once you find out enough to realize that the task is something you don't want to do, you are already obligated. Don't let them put you on the spot—say no right away or insist on complete information to make an informed decision.

Keep in mind that master negotiators know how to use psychology on you—like appealing to ego *("You are the only doctor that could handle this important job")* or guilt *("the company really needs your support right now.")*

CLINICAL VIGNETTE

Dr. Q was a Family doctor who was half way through completing his loan repayment in a Federally Qualified Health

Center working with the underserved. His patients were very challenging due to poverty, low educational levels and health literacy, and required significant time to help them manage their chronic diseases, but he was committed to caring for them, and felt that the work was worthwhile.

At a quarterly physician meeting, administration told the staff that the clinic was in trouble, and that they desperately needed all the doctors to *"just see one or two more patients per day"* for the next month in order to get *"out of the red."* As a salaried physician, there would be no financial incentive for the extra work, but since Dr. Q was concerned about the clinic's future and that of his patients, he redoubled his efforts and, by staying later every day and engaging his team in the mission, he was able to increase his productivity. At the following meeting, Dr. Q was pleased to see from the financial spreadsheet that the clinic's numbers had improved but was surprised when none of the administrators mentioned the team effort that had gone into improving those numbers.

The following quarter, Dr. Q sat in disbelief as the administration repeated nearly verbatim the same mantra they had said before: *"Guys, we are in the red this quarter. We just need everyone to see one or two more patients per day for the next month..."* Dr. Q realized that the *"in the red"* speech happened every quarter and felt completely taken advantage of. He felt ashamed and manipulated, and this took a toll on his work and his health. He even started calling in sick several times per month, which he had never done once in the previous two years.

Try a little negotiation

Doctors have been trained by payers to work for free. Insurance companies don't give us a dime for the time we spend doing paperwork, on the phone with patients or reviewing lab results. So, it's not always in our nature to think about asking to be compensated for our time and labor. We have to change this thinking.

The bottom line: When you are providing a service to your employer by serving on a committee or acting in a leadership capacity, you deserve to be paid for your work. This is especially important when you are working in a productivity model, where any time spent away from actively seeing patients will result in a lower paycheck.

When you are asked to participate in a project or task for your employer, don't be afraid to ask for compensation, and be sure to negotiate for the best deal you can get. If you are asked to go *"above and beyond,"* ask what the additional compensation will be for your work. It doesn't have to be financial—it could be extra vacation days, CME time, etc. Your employer is unlikely to bring up compensation—why would they? The pressure is on you to ask for it.

If your administrator says that they will need to get back to you, don't agree to participate until they do respond—and make sure to get the agreement in writing.

Remember what you are there to do

When considering extra assignments from employers, ask yourself if the job has value, or if it is a token position. If your goals are to move into a leadership position, then serving on a credentialing committee might be a stepping stone for you, but sitting on a birthday celebration committee would be completely out of line with your ideals.

Also, it's essential to ask yourself if additional jobs will impair your clinic work—does this committee take you away from your patients unnecessarily? Will this project negatively impact your financial productivity or your staff/ team relationship? Remember your primary responsibilities. If a request compromises your main reason for existence, then you must say no.

Say no right away

Physicians often dread conflict, and so instead of saying *'no'* immediately, we might try to buy time to come up with an excuse or hope that the asker will forget or ask someone else. Unfortunately, delaying a response just makes it harder, like jumping off a high diving board. Just hold your nose and jump. Remember, you don't have to explain why. Just say no. If you must buy a little time to consider your options, name a concrete time when you will give a definite answer: *"I'll get back to you by Thursday."*

Keep it professional

Saying 'no' in a calm and respectful manner is far better than saying a reluctant 'yes' that ultimately leads you to a point of anger and frustration that leads to unprofessional behavior.

Unfortunately, in our effort to avoid conflict, we may continually say yes when we know we should say 'no'. Now we face an internal struggle of emotion. We are angry and resentful at ourselves for not saying no and at the asker for putting us on the spot. Eventually we are lashing out at everyone around us, deserving or not. We may waste hours trying to escape doing what we agreed to. That causes us to procrastinate on jobs that really need to get done. We may become anxious and depressed. At worst, we may start behaving in ways that administrators love to label as "disruptive"—like yelling, throwing things, and acting in a hostile manner to those around us. And the greatest irony is that these catastrophic results stem from fear of conflict and the inability to say *'no.'*

Unprofessional behavior usually stems from a long buildup of frustration and resentfulness. Work to avoid that behavior by setting boundaries and learning to say 'no' before the pressure builds to a dangerous level.

Remember that you have value. And, generally, your organization needs you more than you need them. So, if they don't respect your limitations, then find a place that will.

ROCK STAR ACTIVITY

Saying 'no'

Think of a situation when you said 'yes' when you should have said 'no.' ____

____

____

What variables led to you saying yes? ________________

____

____

How could you have responded differently? ____________

____

____

What would have changed in your life if you had said 'no?' Would anything bad have happened? ______________

____

____

Practice visualizing yourself in a similar situation saying 'no' and imagine feeling calm and confident in your decision.

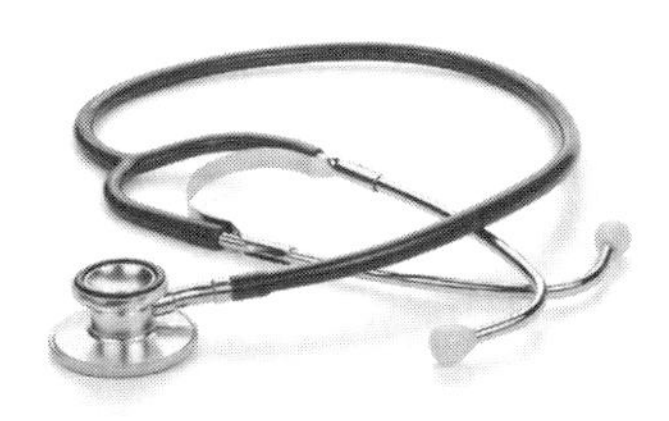

CHAPTER TEN

USE PSYCHOLOGY TO OPTIMIZE WORK EFFICIENCY

One of the biggest complaints that physicians have about office life is spending too many hours at work. In the last chapters, we talked about how physicians tend to overwork, and learned steps that we can take to find work-life balance.

Now, we will focus on psychological steps to optimize our efficiency during work hours so that we can be more productive and get home earlier. We'll start with scheduling.

Although patient care is the part of medicine that most physicians like the best (and the part that earns us our living), studies show that too much time spent with patients is directly correlated with burnout. In fact, beyond an ideal point, each extra hour increases burnout by 2-4%.[xlviii]

The key is to find the "sweet spot:" just the right number of daily patients to apply our trade and make a decent salary, without hitting the level of burnout. Part of accomplishing this is finding and maintaining an intrinsic motivation in what we do (see chapter 7). Another big part, however, is learning to schedule optimally, and knowing how to move patients through our schedule as efficiently as possible.

Office scheduling will vary for every physician, based on each doctor's specialty, practice style, and years of experience. Of course, we also must factor in the practice-specific variables that make seeing patients challenging—the quality of the documentation system, staff support, and patient demographics.

PSYCHOLOGY TIP

The key to office efficiency: Allow the physician to control their own schedule.

Because each practice is so individual, you can only find that scheduling sweet spot by assessing and managing your schedule. This requires consideration of four factors:

1. How long does it take you to provide the care that your patients need?
2. How long do you allow yourself to see those patients?
3. How often do you need a break to recharge?
4. How many daily patient encounters do you need to make enough money to maintain a degree of safety and comfort in your life?

While these four variables need to match up fairly well to avoid physician distress, the reality is that the amount of time that patients require doesn't always match up with the time that we allot ourselves (or are allotted by our employer) to spend with each patient.

Be realistic about your situation. If your patients are complex, if you write long notes, if you have a rotten EHR system, if you have attention deficit disorder or if you have OCD, or if, for whatever reason, you routinely need 30 minutes to see a patient, yet you only schedule yourself fifteen minutes, *you will run behind.*

To help evaluate your office time management, do a time study to see what is really going on in the exam room (use the ROCK STAR ACTIVITY worksheet at the end of the chapter). First, estimate in advance how long you think it will take you to do a task—in this case, to see a patient. Click your timer, then go in and attend to your patient. Once you are finished, come out of the exam room and make an estimation of how long you think you spent with the patient, and write that number down. Now check to see how long you took. Compare the numbers. Are you close or are you way off in your estimations? Did you take longer than you had allotted to see the patient?

Use these time studies as a tool to decide how you want to proceed. Your options are to either change your schedule to match reality or change how you practice to approximate your schedule. If you have flexibility in your schedule (are self-employed or have a sympathetic administrator), change your schedule. If you are locked into an unrealistically rigid schedule, read "How to Be a Rock Star Doctor" for tips to maximize your practice efficiency while you plot your escape to a less toxic practice environment.

MOVING THE OFFICE VISIT ALONG

There are some simple ways to move more quickly through the office visit. Perhaps you need someone to nudge you a bit– one way to stay on time in the exam room is to have your nurse or scribe time your office visits. If you only have time allotted for fifteen minutes, have them remind you at the ten-minute mark, and again when the fifteen minutes is up.

Or, perhaps your office visits are getting delayed due to exam room inefficiencies. The following sections offer techniques to make your life easier and more efficient.

A little preparation goes a long way

In the era of electronic health records, a system failure, where the computers are down for an indefinite amount of time, is catastrophic to your schedule. You can create an analogue back up by having your staff pre-print copies of your last office note for all the patients on tomorrow's schedule. The notes can be placed outside the exam room door for you to quickly peruse before you walk in the room. This serves as a memory jogger for the physician and can also be used as a handout—just jot down any regimen changes and give it to the patient as you conclude the visit. Also, make sure to have any recent labs or tests that were completed since the last visit printed by your staff before you go into the room—this is not something you should be chasing down after you go into the exam room.

Have everything that you will need to care for your patient accessible in the exam room and ideally at your fingertips . That includes resources for patient education, handouts, referral information. Keep them in a computer file to print out when you need them or in a notebook binder.

AUTOMATE AND DELEGATE

We often spend an inordinate amount of time doing repetitive things in the office. Perhaps it's screening kids for attention deficit disorder, ordering lab sets for patients with diabetes or explaining for the one millionth time the difference between viruses and bacterial infections.

Whenever possible, automate your processes. Have all your screening forms nearby and ready to hand to a patient to fill out (bonus points if your nurse did that for you before you walked into the room).

Find or create patient education forms on the most common topics on which you counsel and use them as you educate your patients. This saves you time and allows your patient to take home information for later review. Spend some time upfront with your computer system to create templates for your most common lab order sets, and design generic note templates for various problems that can be edited and personalized for your patients.

Delegate any responsibilities that do not require an MD or DO to your staff. Keep in mind that if your employer expects you to comply with government mandates for meaningful use/ MACRA/ MIPS or whatever acronym is in favor at the time you are reading this book, you are probably going to need a bigger staff. Point out this little pearl to your administration: In 2013, a study showed that to comply with the requirements of the "Patient Centered Medical Home," each physician would require 4.25 'Full Time Equivalent' staff members.[xlix] Remember that if your staff isn't doing the work, that means that *you* are doing it. Probably at home in your pajamas after a long day at the office.

ROCK STAR ACTIVITY

Exam room time study

Patient	Time scheduled	Estimate of how long you think you took	Actual time you took
Jane Doe	15 min	12 min	21 min
Patient	Time scheduled	Estimate of how long you think you took	Actual time you took

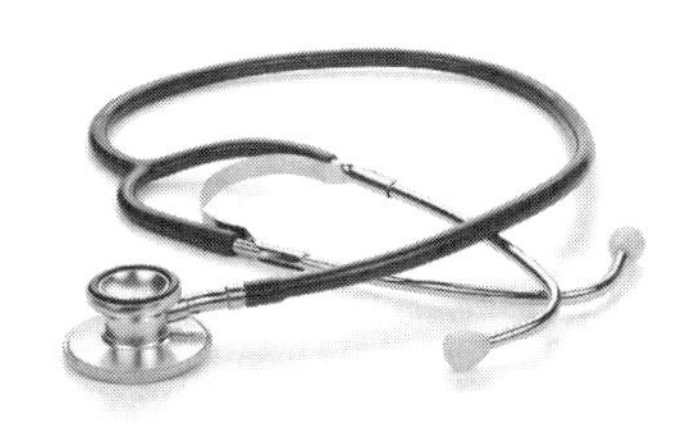

CHAPTER ELEVEN

USE PSYCHOLOGY TO MANAGE A TEAM

As we mentioned, to achieve the payer-required *"patient-centered medical home (PCMH),"* a model that promises more complete patient care, each physician would need 4.25 full-time equivalent (FTE) staff members, compared to the current model of staffing allots just 2.68 FTEs per doc.[1] To paraphrase the movie ***Jaws***, *"You're gonna need a bigger staff."*

Of course, the proponents of PCMH don't give us guidance on how to hire and train these additional staff members, much less how to pay them—which is one of the reasons why many physicians have turned to employed practice, so that a practice manager or administrator can take over this role and just let us be doctors. Or so we hoped.

The reality is that even if we are in employed practice, as physicians, we still have the role of team leader and the responsibility of working with our team members every day. The more involved we are in managing our team, the better our office will function and the happier we will be.

TRAINING YOUR STAFF

Physicians often skip training staff because we are so busy. Instead, we let new staff members learn on the fly or pass them off to other staff members who may not know the correct way of doing things. Unfortunately, this can lead to future problems when an unfollowed policy or procedure leads to a mistake or medical error. This frustrates staff members who need and want clear instructions and guidelines, as well as physicians, who have high expectations for patient care.

New staff members deserve a formal period of training, followed by a review and assessment of their skills. While the physician can delegate this responsibility to an office manager or other individual, he or she should be involved in the process. At a minimum, the physician must ensure that employee training includes the protocols and policies that the physician expects staff to follow, as well as participating in the review process to ensure that each employee is competent to fill the role for which they have been hired.

One of the best ways to do this is to create a policy and procedure manual for your own practice. While each company will have its own manual, rarely does an individual physician take the time to sit down and create a personalized practice manual. While it takes some time on the front end, having a written manual saves endless time down the road. You can then tell staff members to "refer to the manual" for questions, rather than taking your time to look things up yourself.

Include the information that you are always asked—your NPI number, where to find various resources, how to login to the laboratory account, etc. Include your policies on every aspect of the office, from collecting the mail to paying the bills to dealing with biomedical waste. Make it as detailed as possible.

ROCK STAR TIP

Take the time to train your staff up-front to set clear expectations and prevent the development of bad habits.

WORKING WITH STAFF

Sometimes we get frustrated with our staff members when they don't do things the way we would like them to. Recognize every role has its challenges. In fact, the best and busiest physician might have a hard time scheduling appointments and answering phones.

To better understand your staff, spend time with them. Have lunch together occasionally to feel more connected. Just being kind and thoughtful goes a long way. Give praise whenever you see good work and share positive feedback any time you have the opportunity—*"Mrs. Jones told me that your blood draw was the best she ever had—she didn't feel a thing!"*

PSYCHOLOGY TIP

Be lavish with praise when you see something done well: positive reinforcement works! The more specific and detailed the praise, the more weight it carries.

The more connected we are with our staff, the easier it will be to give feedback or suggestions to improve work performance. This can be difficult for physicians, who receive little management training.

The key to providing negative feedback is to:

1. Be present—criticism is most effective when done face-to-face and privately

2. Be sensitive—have empathy and be attuned to what you say, how you say it, and the impact it has.

An artful critique can be one of the most helpful messages that a physician can send a staff member. Done correctly, the staff member will understand what he did wrong and have an optimistic future plan of action. Done incorrectly, the staff member will instead feel helpless, angry, and rebellious.

The art of the critique is to be specific. Pick a significant incident, an event that illustrates a key problem that needs changing or a pattern of deficiency, like the inability to do certain parts of a job well. Focus on the specifics of what was done poorly and how it can be changed. Emphasize the hope that the person can do better and suggest the beginnings of the plan for doing so. It is vitally important that when you tell someone you expect them to *"do better"* or *"work harder"* that you give them a specific way to accomplish this. For example: *"I read your report and it was ok, but I would like you to put in more details about past medical procedures."*

A character attack, calling someone stupid or incompetent, or telling someone they are doing *"a bad job"* without being specific is harmful. This puts them on the defensive, so they are no longer receptive to making change. If a person believes that failure is due to some unchangeable deficit in themselves, they lose hope and stop trying.

DEALING WITH A DIFFICULT EMPLOYEE

Most staff members want to please and improve their performance. Therefore, constructive criticism will be enough to make a positive improvement. However, you may experience a person that you just can't seem to reach, and you may be considering terminating their employment. In this case, there is a technique from psychology that is worth a try before you give up, described by Mark Goulston in the book ***Just Listen*** *(2010)*.[li]

Let's say you have a nurse who has been making several careless mistakes lately. You've had a performance improvement conversation with her, but it hasn't helped. Not only is she still making the same mistakes, but she also seems to have a worse attitude with you.

Begin by letting the person know that you would like to talk with them for a few minutes at the end of the day. Do not meet with them immediately, as you want them to wonder why you want to talk with them. You can indicate that you don't have time right now and that you want to be sure to give them your full attention when you meet. Most likely, the individual will become curious and even somewhat concerned.

To prepare for the meeting, identify a couple of things that you believe the individual finds annoying or difficult about you. Be sure to put yourself in their shoes and try to think like them. For example, *"my nurse is probably disappointed in me for not allowing her more time to practice using the new electronic health record and then expecting her to use it perfectly. She probably hates the way I give her orders abruptly sometimes. I'm sure she must not like it when I speak to her harshly when she asks me to repeat myself."*

As the meeting approaches, the other individual will likely be prepared to receive some criticism and likely be defensive. Point out their expectation, *"I suppose you are expecting me to criticize you like I have in the past. But I am not going to do that. Instead, I have been thinking about some reasons you may be upset with me. I'm guessing that you would never tell me these things because you would be concerned with how I would react."*

Then, tell the person the three things you came up with. When you end, ask them if everything you said was correct and listen to see what the person says.

If they say no, then ask them, *"Then, what are the things that most frustrate you about me?"* Be sure to listen to what they say and repeat them back to ensure that they know that you heard them.

Next, ask them how much those things bother them. When they are done, respond in as genuine of a voice and tone as possible, that you are sorry and will try hard to change your actions in the future.

Now, pause! Pausing can be a great tool to build tension and awkwardness.

After a moment, let the person know that there is nothing else you wanted to talk with them about and thank them for their candor.

If the person inquires as to why you *really* initiated this conversation, say that you know you are not perfect, and you suspect that most people would probably be hesitant to point out your flaws. Also, indicate that you believe that you can do a better job if you know what you are doing wrong.

This approach is going to seem strange and counterproductive at first—why would I throw myself under the bus? I'm not the one with the problem! But as with many psychological techniques that seem counterintuitive at first, it really works.

When you unexpectedly apologize for your actions, you shift the person out of defensive mode and create an emotional response of humility and concern. This can alter the relationship from that of an adversary to one of respect and will often change the individuals attitude and work ethic.

Make sure you chose the correct targets when using this approach, as it works best with people who are trainable—those who need a little push or incentive to shape up. It will not work well with individuals who are entitled or narcissistic because they have an impaired sense of empathy and do not exhibit emotional reciprocity. Using this technique enables us to determine if a staff member is worth keeping. If they respond well, great. If not, it is time to end the relationship.

PSYCHOLOGY TIP

The approach to the difficult employee can also work with other people in your life. Try it with a family member!

THE TROUBLE WITH TEAMS

The only way to comply with the current model of health care with payers' increasing demands for data and box-checking is to utilize a team approach to remove some of the burden from the physician. But rather than using team members to do the burdensome work, many organizations still require physicians to do the most time-consuming elements of data entry, such as CPOE, as discussed in Chapter 6.

Another problem with teams is the development of bystander effect—the probability of getting help is inversely related to the number of people present.[lii] The more team members you have and the more responsibility is diffused, the less sense of accountability any one individual feels. When things go wrong, it can be hard to pinpoint who is responsible and take corrective action.

And, of course, we can't forget about the drama that comes from having multiple different personalities working together in a small area. Sometimes the physician ends up running interference between staff members. That can be distracting and annoying. Physicians may also struggle to find a balance between maintaining professional relationships and developing friendships with staff members, especially when you work closely together every day and learn about your team's personal lives.

CLINICAL VIGNETTE

Dr. H worked for a company that paid very high physician incentives but only low base pay to staff members. Dr. H felt guilty, and as a way of rewarding her team for helping her to earn her high paycheck, she took her staff out for lavish holiday dinners and held all-expense paid annual staff retreats, something that none of the other physicians in her company did. When Dr. H was fired from her job due to her refusal to comply with unethical practices, her entire staff lost their positions as well. Although their job loss was not her fault, the staff was furious

> with Dr. H and blamed her for their unemployment. They began to send her angry Facebook messages and emails—and she had to block them from contacting her. She felt hurt and betrayed with the realization that her staff members were never really her friends.

Sometimes no matter how well a physician works to befriend staff members, there remains a gap in social hierarchy that may be impossible to overcome. There may be a perception that the gap has been bridged, but, in reality, the friendships that develop between employers and staff members tend to be more situational because the relationships are dependent and perceived as obligatory.

Finally, one of the biggest challenges with teams for a physician is that old cliché: *"You are only as strong as your weakest link."* This is particularly problematic in the field of medicine, where the physician holds the ultimate responsibility for patient outcomes but may have little control over the staffing of the practice. If a team member working under your medical license acts in a way that compromises patient safety, the physician bears the ultimate culpability. That is a heavy burden to bear.

A MINIMALIST APPROACH?

One option to avoid managing a team is to make a radical change and cut back to a bare bones approach. The painful truth is that physicians and staff now spend only 1/3 of their time on actual patient care. The rest of our time is being spent on administrative desk work—like checking boxes, filling out forms, and answering insurance demands.

In addition, physicians are spending one to two hours *per night*—time we could be spending with our families, or on our own needs—with our computers, answering the demands of health care payers.[liii]

If you didn't have to deal with insurance companies, government payers, or programs like meaningful use, MACRA, or MIPS, how many staff would you need? If you could write your notes on paper, jot your orders on a script pad, or even just type into a word document, how long would it take you to complete a patient encounter note?

If you didn't have to pay 4.25 FTE staff members, not to mention billing and coders, office managers, and collection companies, what would your overhead be?

Could you afford to make a change? Could you manage to break free?

Hold that thought. We will revisit it in Chapter 19.

ROCK STAR ACTIVITY

Create a physician-specific policy and procedure manual

Create a policy and procedure manual for your personal practice.

Don't feel overwhelmed—you don't have to do it in one day! This can be a work in process—keep it in a computer file and work on it slowly over a period of days to weeks, making note of how your office flows and how you like to function. Don't be afraid to make changes as you go along—this is *your* manual, after all!

Make your policies as clear and as detailed as possible. Once you have a fairly complete manual, print it and place it in binders for each staff member. Ask them to refer to the manual rather than asking you every time they have a question.

As you create your policy manual, take the time to reflect on your medical practice, including your values and goals for yourself and the practice. This is a great opportunity to consider your intrinsic motivators and use them to create a mission statement to include in your office manual.

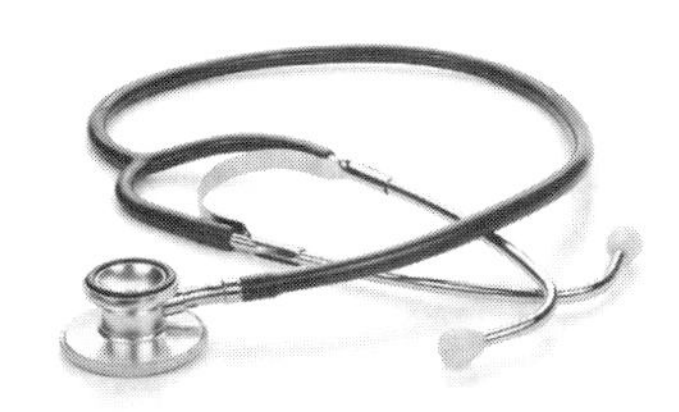

CHAPTER TWELVE

USING PSYCHOLOGY TO IMPROVE PATIENT CARE

The faster you develop strong relationships with your patients, the sooner they will open up about their symptoms and concerns and the more easily you will get to the root of their problems. This in turn helps you to move more efficiently through the office visit. The key to building relationships is developing rapport by learning how to show empathy –that you understand and care. While most doctors do care about their patients, not every physician is naturally good at projecting empathy to make patients *feel* cared about and understood.

There are five simple ways to show empathy. Keep in mind that it is important that all these gestures be perceived by the patient as genuine. That means that you may need to practice these techniques until they feel natural and not forced.

1. Smile. Even if you don't feel happy, smile anyway. When you smile at a patient, even a brief smile, they will automatically smile back. This alone will make them feel more welcome and happier.[liv] So even if you do nothing else, they will already feel better than when they did when they first came in.

ROCK STAR TIP

Practice a small and genuine smile in the mirror until it feels natural. Make sure it comes from the eyes!

2. Engage with the patient in a small physical way. Shake hands. Touch them on the shoulder or elbow.
3. Bond with the patient by making small talk. Ask about the patient's family or hobby, upcoming holiday plans, or even just chat about the weather.
4. Show interest in what the patient has to say. Give the patient your full and complete attention while you are in the exam room. Sit down at their level and look them in the eye. Don't allow interruptions during the visit. Minimize computer contact if you can.
5. Listen to the patient. Avoid interrupting so that they feel that they have been completely heard. Show the patient that you are listening by active listening techniques such as eye contact, leaning forward, and verbal cues. Repeat back what the patient says to you, so they know that you heard and understand them.

PSYCHOLOGY TIP

The key to active listening is making the patient feel heard and understood.

Keep the patient on task

Once you have developed rapport with the patient and have started to explore the patient's medical situation, you may find them wandering off track and onto tangents. At this point, it's ok to gently redirect them back to the current issue. *"I do want to hear about your back pain later but let's get back to the stomach pain that brought you in today."*

Sometimes physicians get overwhelmed when patients give us a laundry list of medical concerns, but we need to remind ourselves that we don't have to (and simply can't!) solve every problem in one visit. However, we *can* listen and acknowledge the patient's concerns so that the patient feels heard, which is sometimes what the patient craves and needs the most.

Make your patients feel heard

1. Simply let them talk. And talk. And talk. In general, most patients won't talk for very long. It may seem like a long time to you at first, because we are used to interrupting with questions or we jump in to redirect or correct a fact. Once the patient stops talking (not just pauses to take a breath, but is really finished with their thought), then you can begin your physician agenda. In many cases, you can skip over 99% of what the patient just said and focus on the clinically relevant part and the patient won't mind, because they were at least able to get their concerns out and they felt heard.

CAVEAT

"The Talker." Every now and then you will come across a patient who literally (and I mean that word in its truest sense) *will not stop talking*. They may be talking to *themselves* as you enter the room. If you ask them questions, they will often ignore them and continue on whatever train of thought they were talking about. They will continue to talk as you type into the computer, print prescriptions, and walk them out to the check-out window. They will still be talking as you walk away, shaking your head. The key to working with these patients is to avoid showing frustration, and instead kindly but firmly redirect them back to the clinical issues that you need to address. With this type of patient, it's ok to interrupt them (if you don't, you will never get out of the room!)—and you can't be subtle. Put your hand out and with a smile, say, *"sorry to interrupt, but I was just checking to see when your last colonoscopy was. Can you remind me?"* Or, "*I hate to interrupt you, but there is some specific information that I really need to get to make sure that I don't miss anything,"* and then without pausing, ask your questions. You'll probably have to do this repeatedly.

2. Another way to help patients feel heard is by listening and then repeating back to the patient what you heard. For example, a patient who comes in for stomach pain begins to describe an additional complaint of musculoskeletal-sounding back pain. The physician allows the patient to explain the pain, then repeats back: *"So you are having pain in your back, that goes down your right leg, but also goes up to your neck and down your left arm too, is that right?"* The patient can then respond: *"Yes, and sometimes the pain also goes down my left leg too."* The physician can validate: *"oh, sometimes it goes down your left leg too… I'm glad you told me that. It must be very uncomfortable, but it sounds like it may be muscular and not dangerous, so I'd like to finish talking about your stomach today, and we can schedule another appointment to talk about your back if it doesn't get better."* Again, the key is repeating back what the patient says when validating so that they feel heard and understood, even if you don't act medically on the information they have offered.

MAKING A CLEAN GETAWAY

Once you have determined how you want to handle your patient's most important clinical issues, it's time to start wrapping up the visit. Perhaps you have ordered some lab tests, prescribed medication or made a referral to another physician. At this point, it's critical to *get out of the exam room.*

The longer you sit in the exam room, the more issues or questions the patient may come up with, which don't always require the physician's attention, like, *"what time does the lab open?"* or *"can you send this prescription to my mail order pharmacy?"* These are generally issues that staff can easily handle.

One way to make a clean exit is to wrap up the appointment by asking the patient: *"Is there anything I haven't asked about today that's important?"* This helps to avoid the "hand-on-the-doorknob" question that drives physicians crazy.

If not, then you can summarize the visit and tell the patient that you are going to bring in a staff member with the patient's prescriptions, orders, etc., and to answer any additional questions about the logistics.

Now, leave the exam room, walk straight into your office or a private area, and *finish your note* (see Chapter 6).

NEEDY PATIENTS

Some patients just seem to take longer than others. We discussed the "talkers" above, but there are also patients who are particularly clingy or needy, and physicians may find it difficult to extricate themselves from the exam room in these cases.

One way to help is to let patients know ahead of time how much time you have for the office visit. Patients don't have any real idea of how long their visits are scheduled for, and doctors rarely share this information. The physician can say: *"We only have fifteen minutes together this morning, and I'm looking forward to hearing what's going on in your life."*

PSYCHOLOGY TIP

Tell patients how much time they have for their visit.

We can also do this when we are getting towards the end of the visit, as a sort of five-minute warning: *"we're about out of time, so let's summarize…"* This helps the patient to start to wrap things up in their mind and allows them to get out any important issues before the visit is over. The more we do this with patients, the more that they will start to get themselves onto a schedule, and they will start to wrap themselves up when the see time ending and will avoid saving the *"big thing"* for the end of the visit.

Some patients don't have good insight into subtleties, so the physician may need to be quite direct about concluding the visit, even to the point of putting his or her hand out and saying, *"We need to stop for today."* Another option is to have a staff member tap on the door at a certain time or send an electronic audible "ding" signal to the computer to message that *"time's up."*

Even though we are setting boundaries with our patients regarding the time that we are giving them, we can also show them that we are not abandoning them by saying something like, *"I'm glad that we're talking about these issues. We don't have the time today that this topic deserves, so I want to schedule another appointment to talk about it in more detail."*

PARTNERING WITH PATIENTS

A key part of office efficiency is developing partnerships with our patients. Our job is to diagnose the patient's condition and recommend a treatment plan, including the known risks, benefits, and alternatives. Our patients' job is to decide whether accept or decline our recommendations. And we need to be ok with that.

PSYCHOLOGY RULE #8:

The doctor should not be working harder than the patient.

It can be hard to be ok with patients when they decline our advice because we feel terrible when patients have bad outcomes. And so, we find ourselves taxing our brains, trying to understand the million different reasons that a patient can't or won't follow a treatment plan. Because we hate to give up. We refuse to accept defeat.

Yet, every day we have patients who choose not to take the medicines we prescribe. Or no-show to the colonoscopy we went through great lengths to set up after explaining how important it was to rule out colon cancer. Or decline the vaccine that will keep them well because they *"don't believe in it."* These are unwinnable situations. And, they can drive us crazy.

But we must remind ourselves that the patient is the one with the problem. Our job is to try our very best to help our patients. But, ultimately, only the patient can take the steps to get better. We can prescribe a medication, make sure that it is on-formulary, spend hours on the phone with the insurance company to get it authorized. But we can't take the medicine for the patient.

Partnering with our patients means involving the patient in the decision-making process for their treatment. Patients must understand their diagnosis and why they are being treated. One way to do this is by dictating the assessment and plan for the office visit in the presence of the patient—that way, they can listen and ask for clarification if they don't understand something.

Another way to help patients to take control of their own health decisions is by helping them to actively think through their choices and come up with their own plan (with your guidance, of course). Rather than lecturing someone on the health consequences of smoking (they already know them) or making them feel guilty about smoking (they already do), ask them to think about what their life would be like if they quit smoking. *"What advantages do you think quitting smoking would bring you?"* Or: *"What sort of things are getting in the way of you quitting smoking?"* When patients think through and identify their own intrinsic motivation, they are much more likely to make lasting changes.

PSYCHOLOGY TIP

This technique is called Motivational Interviewing and can be invaluable to help patients move towards change. The appendix has a list of resources to learn more about this technique.[lv]

It is also very helpful to give patients treatment options, including the option of thinking about our suggestions and then returning to discuss it again after they have had some time to consider. Stay positive and nonjudgmental—*"I know that this can be a lot to take in all at one time. Why don't you take some time to think about it and we can meet again in a week or two?"*

PSYCHOLOGY TIP

To get an accurate idea of how likely your patient is going to participate in your recommendations, simply ask them. For example: *"What percent chance do you think that you will get this colonoscopy done?"* Typically, if their answer is 70% or more, they will follow through. If it is less than 70%, you can be pretty confident they will not comply. Try this on yourself the next time you need to do something that you have been procrastinating or putting off. Sometimes, by simply asking yourself this question, you will alter your answer from 40% to 80% on the spot, and actually complete the task.

Another aspect of partnering with patients involves helping our patients to be accountable for their own care. This means expecting patients to be on-time for appointments, having them bring their medication bottles, asking them to make their own appointments with specialists or to call their own insurance company to find out what medications are on their formulary. Empowered patients work harder at their own health and feel more engaged.

CAVEAT

Doctors tend to be highly intelligent people. We must remember that not everyone has the same capacity for learning as we do. In fact, if the average IQ is 100, that means that 50% of the people that we encounter every day must have an IQ under 100. Do you see where I'm going with this? So, before we get angry when our patient doesn't do what we have asked them to, keep in mind Hanlon's Razor:[lvi] *"Never attribute to malice that which is adequately explained by…,"* well, let's call it a lack of understanding. Or to paraphrase Einstein, *"genius is the ability to express complex ideas or concepts in a manner that the simplest mind can comprehend."* And that's our responsibility.

ROCK STAR TIP

Put patients in charge of their medical records by making them a health care binder and asking them to bring it to every doctor visit. I give a three-ring binder to all my complex patients, with separate tabs for primary care notes, lab results, radiology results, and specialist notes. I punch holes in the patients' reports and place it into the binder at each visit. The patient is responsible to bring the binder to each visit with me and with every doctor they see, especially if they must go to the emergency department.

USING PSYCHOLOGY TO MANAGE CHALLENGING PATIENTS

A major contributor to running late in the office is dealing with challenging patients—the patient who is considered *"unusually difficult"* from the physician's perspective. These patients make up about 15% of patient encounters in primary care and tend to be patients with higher rates of psychiatric conditions and abrasive personality traits. They often report multiple physical symptoms without clear medical explanations, have higher health care utilization, and are more frequently dissatisfied with their medical care.[lvii]

One of the common characteristics to the challenging patient is that they often fear abandonment. Unfortunately, because of the negative emotions that these patients elicit, physicians often *do* try to escape from them, thus fulfilling the patient's greatest anxiety. Fortunately, the use of psychology can ease the stress of managing difficult patients.

The key to coping with difficult patients is using the technique of deep listening and validation of the patient's concerns and scheduling frequent, short follow-up visits.

HOW TO USE DEEP LISTENING AND VALIDATION

Deep listening allows the clinician to overcome conflict, and involves three elements:

1. showing empathy
2. mirroring of emotions, or relating your understanding of how the patient is feeling
3. avoid trying to fix or solve the problem (in other words, shut up and be patient).

Part of the problem with strong emotions is that they are controlled by the primitive and mammalian brain, which is responsible for core, raw emotions and our fight-or-flight response, rather than our more advanced neocortex, or *"human"* brain. When we are experiencing a strong emotional state, such as anger, sadness or fear, the mammalian brain becomes active and takes control over the human brain. It then supersedes our higher order brain functions of empathy and advanced thinking.

In strong emotional states, our amygdala becomes overstimulated, locking us into our mammalian brain and preventing us from accessing our higher order brain function. Daniel Goleman, in his book *Emotional*

Intelligence (1995), termed this state *"amygdala hijacking."*[lviii] That's why someone in a strong emotional state may respond poorly to directions, commands, or suggestions. For instance, if you say to an angry person *"Stop yelling,"* they may yell back, *"I'm not yelling!"*

The key to overcoming amygdala hijacking is the technique of emotional mirroring. Mirroring is an automatic process that we do regularly without thinking and may be controlled by cells in our brain called mirror neurons, which fire constantly as we are engaging with another person.[lix]

For example, when we are walking with a friend, we will find our paces synchronizing naturally. Or, we may find ourselves nodding or tapping along to music playing in concert with a person sitting across the room. In fact, mirroring is so powerful that smiling at a stranger will evoke an automatic smile in return or watching someone hit their finger with a hammer will evoke a grimace from a bystander.

Emotional mirroring can be as simple as repeating back and validating the patient's emotional state. It's an excellent tool to defuse an emotionally charged situation.

So, if a physician is faced with an emotionally charged individual, perhaps someone who is angry or extremely anxious, she can take several steps to defuse the situation.

1. First, identify the emotional state based on what the patient is saying, as well as by the nonverbal cues that the patient is showing (facial expressions, gestures, mannerisms). In this case, we will use an example of a patient who seems tense and stressed. He has his arms crossed, he is jiggling his foot, and is breathing rapidly.
2. Next, practice emotional mirroring: Simply state to the patient how you believe he is feeling.

   Doctor: *"You seem to be very stressed today."* Ask them if you are correct. *"Is that right?"* Note that people often get defensive when you use words like anxious, and tend to respond better to words like stressed, tense, worried, or nervous.

3. If you are correct, continue to mirror the patient's emotions.

   Patient: *"Yes, I am very stressed. I'm worried about my test results."*
   Doctor, mirroring and validating: *"You are worried about your test results. I can imagine that must be exhausting."*

4. If you are not correct, ask them how they are feeling and then proceed to mirror the emotional state they identify.

   Patient: *"No, I'm not stressed."*
   Doctor: (in a genuine and compassionate tone—being genuine is vital to the success of this technique) *"Oh, then, how are you feeling?"*
   Patient: *"Well, I'm pissed off!"*
   Doctor, mirroring: *"Oh! So, you are feeling pissed off."*
   Patient: *"Yes! I'm pissed off because I've been waiting for an hour!"*
   Doctor, mirroring and validating: *"Wow, you have been waiting for an hour. I can see how upsetting and irritating that must be for you to have to wait so long. I bet you're feeling pretty annoyed and impatient with me right now."*

Believe it or not, at this point the patient will likely deescalate and ally to you saying, *"no, I know you are busy, you know your stuff, that's why I want to see you over someone else, so I don't mind waiting."* If not, continue to step 5.

5. Allow the patient to continue to talk, listening, mirroring, and validating until you hear an audible exhale. This signals that a transition has occurred from the mammal brain to the human brain, and the patient is ready to move forward.

Do not try to address the person's problem until they invite you to offer feedback, saying something like, *"so, what do you think?"* or, *"well, are you going to tell me about my results?"* This type of statement signals that the person has now moved past being stuck in an emotional state and is beginning to use higher order thinking, where problem solving occurs.

Remember, you are not telling the patient that they are right nor do you have to agree with them! You are simply letting them know that you understand their emotional state and belief set at that moment.

You can learn more about emotional mirroring through the resources at the end of the book, or work with a psychologist trained in this technique. It really works.

FREQUENT FOLLOW-UP

One of the most important elements of managing emotionally challenging patients is to schedule frequent follow-up visits. Patients with psychosocial stress often have a multitude of symptoms and complaints, which can never be dealt with in one visit. Encourage patients to discuss their top one or two concerns today and then schedule an appointment for the near future to discuss the rest. That helps you to keep running on time.

Additionally, patients considered difficult by doctors often fear abandonment. That makes them engage in behaviors like frequent phone calls and drop-by visits that can create chaos. Frequent scheduled visits provide patients with reassurance and improves the therapeutic relationship. And remember that an emergency on their part does not necessarily constitute an emergency on yours!

THE CHALLENGE OF CONTROLLED SUBSTANCES

Physicians face dilemmas every day when it comes to controlled substances. On the one hand, we feel an obligation to treat pain and anxiety and to help our patients. Yet, we are deeply concerned about the dangers of medication dependence and abuse, in particular as we deal with our present opioid crisis. The situation is compounded by intense patient pressure that includes techniques of manipulation *("I've tried everything; this is the only thing that works!")*, guilt *("are you just going to let me suffer, doctor?")*, threats *("If you don't give it to me, I'm going to have to get it off the streets")*, and ego-manipulation (*"But Dr. X always prescribed this for me."*.

CLINICAL VIGNETTE

Dr. G was a new Family Medicine graduate who was trained during the *"Pain is the 5th Vital Sign"* era. She was a very kind-hearted doctor, with a tendency to believe her patients implicitly. When they told her that their pain was uncontrolled, she increased their opioid doses and transitioned them to long acting opioids, just as she had been taught in residency. Unfortunately, word got around in the small town where she practiced that she was a liberal prescriber. Soon her waiting room was full of sad stories of chronic pain. Some of Dr. G's patients began to warn her that other patients were selling their medications on the street, but she didn't believe it, because she was spending a great deal of energy following all the guidelines for drug testing and pain contracts and checking databases. Eventually a patient stole a prescription pad from the office. Dr. G made a police report, resulting in an extensive court case which took up even more of her time. Dr. G began to feel depressed and overwhelmed dealing with chronic pain patients.

While most physicians are well-versed in the *"tells"* of drug seeking patients, we don't always get much instruction on how best to help these patients while reducing our own emotional angst. Fortunately, there are psychological techniques that we can use to show empathy towards patients while also providing them with the best medical care and maintaining our own sanity.

Create an office policy on controlled substances

One of the best defenses against emotionally manipulative patients is to create an office policy and to enforce it strictly. For example, the Drug Enforcement Agency points out that one of the characteristics of patients with drug abuse issues are unusual requests that should automatically raise a red flag, such as the need to be *"seen right away,"* calling or coming in after regular hours, a new patient who states he/she is traveling through town, visiting friends or relatives, or a request for a replacement prescription for one that has been lost or stolen.[lx]

An easy way to avoid these types of situations is to institute an office policy that states that controlled substances are never prescribed at the initial visit for a new patient nor outside of regular office hours nor are these types of prescriptions replaceable regardless of reason—the dog ate the prescription, the pills fell into the sink, etc. This is our office policy, period. Sometimes it is easier to *"blame"* it on the office policy than to say that it is your policy.

Another office policy is to routinely check your state prescription database for every patient for whom you are considering prescribing a controlled substance. This isn't a judgment of the patient—it's a policy that you perform on every single patient for the sake of safety and allows you to verify that the patient hasn't received similar prescriptions from other physicians recently and that there is no evident history of misuse. Everyone has their ID checked when buying alcohol at the grocery store—checking a database is not an accusation of guilt—it's just a good policy for safety.

De-escalate with emotional mirroring

Patients who are suffering physical or emotional pain are often highly emotionally charged. Part of the problem is that patients with chronic illness or pain have trouble *not* thinking about their symptoms, a powerful psychiatric phenomenon in which the symptoms become intensified over time, leading to cognitive distortions. For example, a person with chronic pain or depression who doesn't sleep well may say: *"I haven't slept in a month"* and they believe their exaggeration. Even though we know logically that a person cannot go a month without sleeping, the cognitive distortion leads a person to believe something that is illogical—in this case, they truly *believe* that they haven't slept for a month.

Rather than challenging the patient's cognitive distortion (because they simply will not believe you, no matter what proof you give), instead try emotional mirroring and empathy. This builds rapport and makes the patient more open to considering alternatives that you will offer to the controlled medication that they want.

> Patient: *"I need Xanax. I haven't slept in a month."*
>
> Doctor: *"You haven't slept in a month? You must be exhausted."*

Spend time exploring the patient's symptoms and their emotional state surrounding the symptoms. Reflect what they say to confirm that you do *"get"* it. Try to gather as many details about the patient's symptoms as possible. In particular, what is the link between their emotional and physical response.

> Patient: *"I need Xanax for my panic attacks. It is the only thing that works."*
> Doctor: *"How long does it take the Xanax to work for you?"*
>
> Patient: *"It works so well, like within seconds I feel so much better, I can breathe."*

Doctor: *"The Xanax works in seconds. It makes you feel much better when you take it."*

Patient: (with relief) *"Yes, you understand."*

Doctor: *"I understand that it makes you feel better."* (pause, and wait for patient response)

Patient: *"Yes, it so does!"*

Doctor: *"But Xanax is making you feel better because your mind is expecting to feel better from it. The medicine isn't even working yet within seconds—it takes at least 20 minutes to start working. This is good news—it means that we should be able to help you feel better without having to take a pill."*

Give options

Once you build a therapeutic relationship with the patient by deep listening, you can start to work on a treatment plan. Rather than simply saying *'no'* right off the bat to the patient's requested medication, start on a positive by giving some alternatives. *"I have some suggestions for other medications that I think would work even better for you and would be much safer."*

In many cases, the patient is going to be on the defensive and quick to respond that they have already tried x, y, and z. Review each medication option in detail with the patient and ask them specifically what problems the medication gave them, including the circumstances of the side effects. If you find a medication that the patient hasn't already tried, or is open to trying, great! If not, keep going down your list of options until you run dry. If the patient insists that they have tried and failed *every single medication* except their drug of choice, and you definitely don't think that they should be on the medication they want, then you will need to be direct: *"I understand that Xanax* is the medication that you feel that you need, however, because of the other medications that you take, I do not think* *that Xanax is in your best interest, and I am not going to prescribe it for you. I do understand that you are suffering. So, I would really like to re-try one of the other medications that I mentioned before. Because maybe this time will be different for you, and I think it can help this time. We can start it at a lower dose and follow up very closely to see how you respond." (*Author's Note: The use of Xanax here is an example in this scenario only. In some cases, alprazolam may be medically appropriate.)*

Keep the patient's best interest in mind and stay strong

Remember, as the physician, you are in charge. You are the expert. WebMD may make the patient think that they are the expert, but patients don't always know what they need. What they think they need doesn't make it true. This goes for pain medications, antibiotics, unnecessary MRIs, you name it.

We worry about our patients getting upset, complaining about us or firing us as doctors if we say no, but in general, patients expect doctors to be confident and won't be offended if *'no'* comes across the right way, by showing that you are listening, and you do understand them. What matters is that you are confident and that you trust your own judgment.

Don't be wishy-washy or uncertain when you say no. When we don't seem confident, patients can tell that if they keep nagging, we will give in. And, sometimes physicians find dealing with patients with chronic pain or anxiety so exhausting that we do just give in and write the prescription to *"get it over with"* and move on to our next patient.

Unfortunately, when we do this, we are training our patients that the more they ask us, the more likely we are to give in to what they want. In fact, behavioral psychology shows that intermittent reinforcement is the worst thing that we can possibly do. When we give in to patient pressure from time to time (intermittent reinforcement), we create something called *"resistance to extinction"* in that patient.[lxi] In other words, when we give in to the patient sometimes, it becomes harder for the patient to resist the behavior. And they are more likely to continue to ask for the medication that we don't want them to have. It is far better to train our patients from the beginning that when the medication that they want is not in their best interest, we will stay firm in refusing to prescribe it because we really do care about them and don't want to see them harmed.

We must also educate our patients about the potential harms of medications. For example, many patients don't realize that mixing benzodiazepines and opioids, even at low doses, can be lethal. Or patients may be in denial about their substance abuse problems. We need to be able to have the conversation with our patients where we can say to them: *"I'm really worried about you."* Sometimes showing a patient their spreadsheet from the prescription database where they have been receiving multiple prescriptions from different doctors and pharmacies can help them to confront the reality of their substance abuse problem.

While physicians often dread confrontation, we must be open and honest with our patients about the dangers of misusing medications. In fact, our patients may finally be ready to get help when provided with the opportunity in a supportive environment.

Responding to threats

As we discussed above, patients with addictions and chronic pain are often emotionally charged. Sometimes they lash out with verbal abuse, including threats: *"I'm going to tell everyone what an uncaring doctor you are!"* or *"I'm going to post on all the doctor review sites that they shouldn't come to this practice."* Sometimes they even threaten themselves: *"If you don't prescribe my pain medication, I'm going to have to find it on the street."*

The best way to respond to a threat is to acknowledge it and show empathy. *"If I don't prescribe this pain medication, you are telling me that you will get it from the street. I'm hoping that you won't feel the need to do that if you take these other steps that I have suggested."* Often patients will backtrack from their statements when their *"primitive"* brain is no longer in command.

In some cases, threats cannot be tolerated. If a patient is threatening your safety or that of your staff, report them to the authorities immediately and dismiss them from your practice. Don't feel guilty because not acting simply enables the patient and reinforces their negative behaviors.

CLINICAL VIGNETTE

Dr. R. was caring for a young man with severe brain damage from an auto accident. When she declined to sign a paper to authorize the return of his driver's license, he became enraged. He left her office and went to his physical therapist appointment, where he told his physical therapist *"I'm going to get a gun, go to Dr. R's office and kill her."* The therapist called Dr. R, who was shaken. She reported the threat to the Sheriff's department, and the patient was transferred to the local psychiatric crisis center for treatment.

Be aware of your emotions

Some patients with addiction issues can be master manipulators. They use charm, charisma, and guilt to get what they want out of those around them, including their physicians. These patients are often very likeable and can spin a tale that can leave even the most seasoned doctor feeling betrayed when they discover that they were lied to.

We feel guilty when we cannot alleviate patient suffering, and patients sometimes prey upon that guilt: *"Can't you see that I'm hurting?"* We must also be willing to sacrifice our ego when patients compare us to other physicians: *"my old doctor always prescribed this medication for me, and it worked great with no side effects—why won't you?"*

Finally, we must avoid our urge to *"people please"* and battle the discomfort we feel when we disappoint our patients. We must remind ourselves that acting in the patient's best interest doesn't always mean doing exactly what the patient wants. Also, realize that what the patient thinks is in their best interest may well be inaccurate.

USE YOUR PSYCHOLOGIST COLLEAGUES

While physicians can help patients with many psychosocial issues, there is no substitute for counseling with a licensed mental health professional as part of a comprehensive treatment plan. We should liberally refer our difficult patients to an excellent psychologist to help them deal with their emotional and physical health problems, including chronic pain, which has been shown to benefit from CBT.[lxii] This not only helps our patients, but also frees up our time for our other patients.

As physicians, we can also work personally with a psychologist to learn tools and techniques that help us to manage our difficult patients, such as learning more about mirroring and validation, how to read body language, and how to help our patients cope with psychological stressors, especially if our patients won't go to the psychologist themselves.

PSYCHOLOGY RULE #9

The people who really need to go to the psychologist won't go. That's why the rest of us have to.

Keep this in mind: According to the 2016 National Survey on Drug Use and Health, only about half of adults in the United States with a serious mental illness receive treatment for their mental health problem.[lxiii]

While part of this may be due to lack of treatment availability, a big cause is something called anosognosia—the lack of insight into the need for treatment. This condition is not simply denial but is a true inability to recognize the symptoms of mental illness, caused by a neurologic deficit that is associated with structural brain changes in people with serious mental illness. Working with these patients can present a very difficult challenge to physicians, especially those of us without a strong psychiatric background. And we will need help and support from our colleagues.

ROCK STAR TIP

Reduce the stigma of seeing a psychologist by putting it this way: Of *course,* I go to a psychologist; do you have any idea what I *do* all day?"

ROCK STAR ACTIVITY

Practice emotional mirroring and validation

Follow these steps: Ask an open-ended question. Listen carefully to the response and try to reflect or mirror back what the person said in your own words, and then respond in a validating or empathetic way.

When done correctly, this practice should strengthen your patient relationships and make for a more effective office visit. If you aren't seeing positive results, schedule an appointment with a psychologist to watch your technique and give you pointers.

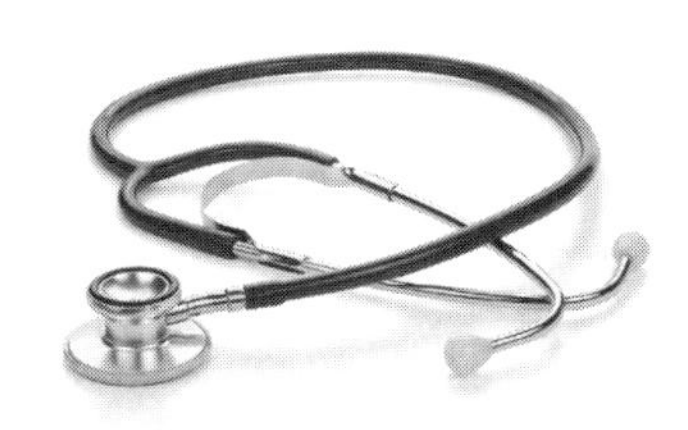

CHAPTER THIRTEEN

MENTAL HEALTH—THE IMPACT OF NEGATIVE THINKING ON MOOD

"Where there is ruin, there is hope for a treasure."
- Rumi

Physicians, just like the patients we serve, suffer with mental health conditions, including depression, anxiety, and substance abuse disorders. While depression rates among practicing male physicians seems to be about the same as in the general population, around 12 to 13 percent, [lxiv] it is higher among women at 19.5%,[lxv] and has been found to be much higher among medical students and residents.[lxvi]

In the next three sections, we will examine the major emotional stressors of physicians and include a plan of attack to deal with each, including tools for colleagues to help their peers cope most effectively with emotional stress. Because this book focuses on psychology, we will limit recommendations to non-pharmaceutical treatments. And we urge anyone with serious symptoms to consult with their physician. In many cases, medication therapy may be appropriate and extremely beneficial.

MOOD ISSUES AND DEPRESSION

The increased risk of depression in physicians, particularly in women and medical students and residents, may be partially explained by role strain—the high social expectation and idealization placed on individuals playing the "role" of doctor. The physician is expected to function at maximal competence at all times. Not doing so leads to personal and social *"disapprobation."*[lxvii] To borrow the phrase from the Apollo mission, *"failure is not an option."* And yet, as human beings, failure is inevitable.

The societal and internal pressure of this unrealistic and impossible physician ideal can be so powerful that the physician, particularly during the early training phase, will overwork and sacrifice personal needs to try to achieve this goal, but will find that there is no way to keep up. Failures must and will occur. Now we face an internal conflict: do we learn to accept our limitations? Or, do we turn towards destructive behavior—excessive working, spousal neglect, alcohol or drug use—in an effort to continue to push towards an impossible ideal?

The role strain conflict is particularly powerful for women, who may juggle the roles of spouse and mother with that of physician. Again, the harder she applies herself to one role, the more she faces failures in another. This is particularly difficult for physicians, who are *"not supposed"* to fail.

PSYCHOLOGY TIP

Depression is often linked to role strain conflict—the balance between roles as physician with roles as spouse, parent, etc. Identifying our roles and accepting our limitations in those roles can be a first step to addressing depression. Further, acknowledging

the importance of each role and its individual significance helps to create and maintain a sense of balance.

The risk of depression is also associated with other challenges that physicians face in our careers: lack of sleep, dealing with death, making mistakes, 24-hour responsibility, and self-criticism, as well as difficult relationships with coworkers and patients.[lxviii]

Depression increases the risk of suicide. And studies have shown that physicians have higher suicide rates than the general population, with 400 physicians per year dying by suicide.[lxix] While men physicians have modestly higher rates of suicide, women have much higher rates than the general population.[lxx]

Physicians with underlying depression, bipolar disorder, alcohol abuse, and substance abuse are at increased risk for suicide.[lxxi] Suicide is a behavior that stems from an irrational thought process. Our internal safety mechanisms, such as the instinct for self-preservation, are turned off and replaced with a desire to escape a distorted perception of reality. In other words, when we are having suicidal thoughts, we are simply not in our right mind at that present moment.

The development of suicidal thoughts can happen over time from progressive depression. Mental health treatment of depression may be able to prevent the decompensation towards suicidal intent.

Suicide may also be provoked by a sudden traumatic event which triggers an intense sense of helplessness and hopelessness. If a physician is receiving adequate mental health care at the time of the serious event, they may have improved emotional and cognitive resilience to withstand the impact of the trauma.

While timely mental health care may prevent suicides, physicians are not getting help when they need it. Studies show that most physicians who commit suicide were not receiving mental health treatment at the time of their death.[lxxii]

What can we do to get better?

Fortunately, we live in a time when treatment for depression and other mental health conditions is significantly safer and more effective than ever. And yet, as mentioned above, most physicians who ultimately took their own lives were not receiving treatment when they died. Why is this?

It is extremely difficult for physicians to reach out for help with anything, but it is especially hard for us to seek help for mental health issues. One reason for our reluctance is that it is particularly difficult for us to acknowledge our problems because we are perfectionists and fear showing weakness.

Another reason that physicians fail to get help for mental health issues is because of perceived or real threats to our careers if we acknowledge such an issue. For example, in a survey of surgeons, even though 1 in 16 had experienced suicidal thoughts, only 26% of those affected sought psychological help, partially because they worried that receiving treatment could affect their medical licensure.[lxxiii]

In addition to concerns over loss of licensure, physicians also fear the stigma associated with using mental health services, fear of documentation on our record, and fear of an unwanted intervention for seeking help for mental health issues.[lxxiv]

Acknowledging the need for help

First, realize that you are not alone. When we are down or depressed, we often feel isolated and alone in our suffering. Just being aware of the statistics on physician depression can demonstrate that many others experience the same difficulties.

Acknowledge that asking for help is not a sign of weakness. In fact, it takes more courage to ask for help than it does to suffer in silence. And getting help makes us better and stronger.

Accept that feeling depressed is not your fault or a personal shortcoming. You've probably given this lecture to your patients a thousand times. *"You wouldn't blame a child with diabetes for needing insulin, would you? So why do you blame yourself when you need help with mental health issues?"*

Get past the fear of stigma and career threat. While these concerns may be legitimate, we must acknowledge that failure to seek help will result in far worse problems with licensure. That could mean losing our medical license permanently if mental health problems escalate into behaviors that compromise patient safety. Also, be aware that you may be able to obtain mental health assistance while avoiding some of the stigma and documentation issues that physicians fear.

Finding help

A first step to finding help with mental health issues is to talk with a trusted colleague or your personal physician and get a referral to an excellent psychologist, and if needed, a psychiatrist. While the Mental Health Parity Act, updated by George W. Bush in 2009, requires health insurance companies to provide mental health coverage at the same level as physical health benefits, some physicians may prefer not to use their health insurance to pay for mental health care due to concerns over privacy issues. In this case, most psychologists are willing to work with patients on a fee-for-service basis.

PSYCHOLOGY TIP

The options for mental health care providers can be confusing. Like *"medical doctor,"* *"psychologist"* is a legal term. The title *"psychologist"* indicates that the individual has a doctoral degree (PhD or PsyD), has completed internship and post-doctoral

training, and has passed both national and state examinations. Other mental health providers such as licensed counselors (LMHC, LMHT) and clinical social workers (LCSW) do not have the same requirements.

Some county medical societies now provide confidential psychology services as a membership benefit under a Physician Wellness program. The Lane County Medical Society in Oregon was the first county medical society to create a physician wellness program in 2012, with the goal of helping physicians *"find the balance between the demands of their work and personal lives."*[lxxv] Many other counties are developing similar programs. These programs usually offer 6-8 free annual sessions with a psychologist that are unreported and confidential. (See Appendix D for a list of county Physician Wellness Programs or contact your local county medical society to see if they have a program or plan to create one).

To get the best results, physicians must work with a trained clinician in a structured fashion. In other words, we must avoid treating ourselves or using friends or colleagues informally for medical care. Physicians have a tendency to try to self-diagnose and self-medicate, which obviously is less objective. Once we enter professional treatment, we often try to direct our own care, which our colleagues may allow, as they subconsciously identify with the physician-patient, minimizing the extent of illness.[lxxvi] Unfortunately, being a *"special patient"* may result in inferior care.[lxxvii] That's why it is vital for your optimal benefit to create a truly objective therapeutic relationship with a mental health professional.

PSYCHOTHERAPY WORKS

Skeptical about working with a psychologist? Don't be!

First, let's clarify that there is a big difference between sitting down for a few sessions with a counselor or a pastor or your best friend for *"talk therapy"* and working with a licensed psychologist experienced in cognitive behavioral therapy (CBT). CBT is a goal directed, empirically validated treatment approach to multiple serious psychologic conditions.[lxviii] And it works.

Multiple studies have shown that CBT can significantly improve our thinking patterns, beliefs, attitudes, emotional states, and behaviors.[lxxix] What's more, these changes can persist over time.[lxxx] Functional brain scans have revealed normalization in brain activity during psychotherapy treatments, including changes in our brain circuitry such as calming effects in the parts of our brain that control the symptoms of depression and anxiety.[lxxxi]

Studies also show that CBT for depression can result in something called *"sudden gains,"* a large improvement in symptoms of up to 50% in just a single between-session interval, which lasted a full eighteen months.[lxxxii]

Take care of yourself

Physicians are notorious for *"presenteeism"*—coming into work not only when we are exhausted or sick, but even when we are severely depressed.[lxxxiii] We may do this out of sense of responsibility and irreplaceability, but sometimes we do it because of a dysfunctional strategy to manage depression. Work can act as a sense of structure and routine that sometimes keeps us going and distracts our mind temporarily from negative thoughts. However, lack of sleep, protracted work hours, and illness are associated with worsening depression, making this type of behavior counterproductive.

Part of self-care for depression, as well as other emotional stressors, includes managing our physical needs of adequate sleep, nutrition, exercise, recreation, and social activities.

CLINICAL VIGNETTE

> Dr. J was a successful, well-liked specialist in his early 50s with a thriving out-patient and hospital practice. He appeared at many medical society meetings with his beautiful wife on his arm and a ready smile on his face. When he died suddenly by suicide, the medical community was shocked and bewildered. Was there anything that anyone could have done to prevent this horrific outcome?

The loss of someone we know by suicide is extremely distressing. Besides the pain of losing someone from our lives, we often ask ourselves if there was anything that we could have done to have helped, or if there was something that we missed, some sign or signal.

Sadly, there are often no outward signs of an impending suicide. People who go on to demonstrate suicidal behaviors often present themselves to the outside world with a mask that "everything is alright." They tend to hide their negative thoughts and feelings from others, which is why suicide often comes as such a shock.

However, if we can identify our colleagues who are suffering with depression or emotional stress before their thinking becomes severely impaired, we can help empower them to acknowledge and share their negative feelings. This is critical to preventing dysfunctional thinking that can lead to a later break with reality and result in suicide.

HOW TO RECOGNIZE A PHYSICIAN IN NEED

First, understand that while the signs of physician distress may be present, we may not always be aware of them. The truth is that, as human beings, we sometimes only see what we expect to see or what we want to see. By being aware of our own cognitive biases, we can look deeper for the signs of a colleague in need.

Sometimes we fail to see signs of depression because it causes us emotional pain to see this in people we care about or admire.[lxxxiv] Often we assume that behavior changes stem from stress or overwork, because we are uncomfortable with the thought of a distressed colleague. However, failure to acknowledge the signs of depression does a disservice to our fellow physicians. And so, we must acknowledge our own discomfort and forge ahead.

One common sign of physicians in distress is a change in their typical patterns of behavior. For example, a physician who is usually cheerful suddenly becomes irritable and cranky. Or a person who is always on time is now suddenly rushed and last minute, or an organized person is now constantly misplacing things. Any change in typical persona can signal a problem.

Another sign of distress is physician isolation from others. This can sometimes manifest as last-minute cancellations. The physician may agree to attend events or activities, then cancel at the last minute when something unexpectedly *"comes up"* every time. They may withdraw from interacting with friends or colleagues, which we may sometimes miss because we take it personally (*"why isn't Dr. Smith talking to me? Did I do something wrong?"*). They may come in late or exceptionally early to work to avoid small talk with colleagues or time with family. Another sign of isolation is ignoring or failing to respond to texts, phone calls, or emails.

PSYCHOLOGY TIP

Signs of physician distress include a change in usual pattern of behavior and isolation from others.

Finally, doctors dealing with depression may experience any of the typical anhedonia symptoms we observe with our patients—lack of interest in activities they used to enjoy. They may report fatigue, somatic or physical complaints, appetite or weight changes or be short-tempered or irritable.

How to respond

Many times, physicians may notice a colleague in distress, but fail to act due to a variety of concerns. Some refer to this as a *"conspiracy of silence,"* in which our natural tendency is to rationalize or ignore a colleague's impairment.[lxxxv] We may fail to act because we assume that our colleagues will be able to work out their problems on their own, because we fear stigmatizing our fellow physicians or because we assume that someone else will address the situation. We may not reach out because we don't know what resources are available or what to do if a colleague does share mental health issues. We may also fail to act because we are uncomfortable with feelings and emotions.

STEPS TO INTERACTING WITH DISTRESSED COLLEAGUES

If your gut says that something is wrong with a colleague, believe it. If you hear others talking about a physician acting unusual, address the concerns with the physician directly. Don't assume that someone else will step up, as often no one will—a phenomenon called *"bystander effect"* where everyone assumes that someone else will take charge, and no one actually does anything.

Find a time when the physician is not rushed and when you have enough time to give your complete attention. The end of the day, when they have finished with patient care and are wrapping up paperwork is often a good time. Pick a private area, like the physician's office.

Start by asking in a general way: *"How are you?"* or *"I notice that you seem to be stressed lately—is everything ok?"* As they answer, watch them carefully for their facial expression and body language, and listen to their tone of voice.

Because opening up feels like a weakness to many physicians, they will often respond with *"Everything's fine,"* but you may see certain cues to indicate that the physician is not fine, such as a head shake from side to side after answering or ending the statement in a questioning tone, as if they are trying to convince themselves.

It can be difficult for a depressed physician to even believe that a colleague really cares because of the cognitive distortions associated with depression. This is where the use of empathy can be helpful to really show that we are concerned. We can respond to the answer of the physician that *"everything's fine"* by saying: *"Everything's fine? OK, I just feel like something is off and I was worried about you."* This lets the physician know that we really do want the answer to how they are doing, and not just a token reply.

If the physician does start to open up or give hints as to their emotional distress, be prepared to listen and show empathy. But no matter what, don't start trying to problem solve!

WHAT DO I MEAN BY THIS?

Often when a physician does start to open up about emotional stress, they do it in a more general and *"safe"* way, like listing the problems that they are facing at work. For example: *"Well, yeah, I guess I am a little stressed. It's just that this damn EHR system is really beating me down. And they expect me to see too many patients in one day. And my nurse just quit, and they gave me someone new, and she has no idea what she is doing..."* and so on. While these problems are real, they may only be a small part of the general emotional distress that the physician is experiencing.

Our natural inclination may be to try to start problem solving: *"OK, well, let's strategize on ways to work more effectively with the EHR. And maybe we can talk to administration about finding you a different nurse,"* but this isn't actually addressing the root of the problem. The physician needs to be able to start opening up and sharing emotions, but when you shift into *"problem solving"* mode, you actually shut down the flow of emotion. We need to allow the physician the opportunity to continue to express feelings and emotions, and validate those feelings, without trying to "fix" them.

This is tough! When others share their feelings, we get uncomfortable. We feel helpless. We want to fix things. We want to fix the emotion. But we can't fix feelings, and we don't have to. The feeling isn't broken. The feeling just *is*.

Rather than problem solving, simply allow the physician to continue to share feelings and validate those emotions. Listen to the *"feeling"* words or descriptors that the physician says, and repeat them back, or use a synonym.

If the physician says, *"I'm just totally wiped out with all this extra work,"* you can respond: *"I'm guessing you feel like you're never going to get through it all."*

You will know if you are getting it right if the physician responds in an accepting way, in agreement, and continues talking and sharing. If you are getting their feeling wrong, they will get defensive—sometimes this will happen even when you use the same word they used, but it wasn't exactly what they meant.

Encourage professional help

Once a colleague has started to open up about concerns, this is a good opportunity to encourage them to talk to a professional. It is our responsibility to reduce the stigma towards mental health care. Say something like *"You're going through a tough time—take advantage of the resources out there."* Remind them that it's not a weakness to ask for help, and that it takes more courage to accept help. Getting help makes you a better person and a better physician.

PSYCHOLOGY RULE #10

The better we care for ourselves, the better we can care for others.

Even if the physician isn't ready to accept a referral for further help right now, just starting the conversation may open the door for future consideration. It also lets the physician know that you are truly concerned and available if they need to talk in the future.

SUBSTANCE ABUSE

Estimates of substance abuse indicate that about 15% of physicians will be impaired at some point in their careers, about on average with the general population.[lxxxvi] However, women seem to be at higher risk for alcohol abuse, with 21.4% of women physicians meeting diagnostic criteria in one study, compared to 12.9% of men physicians.[lxxxvii] Physicians are also at higher risk of self-medicating with opioids and benzodiazepines.[lxxxviii]

It can be difficult to recognize the symptoms of substance abuse, as they can be similar to those of depression. Also, unusual behavior in physicians associated with substance abuse is sometimes excused as *"eccentric"* behavior or blamed on overwork or stress. Just as with working with a depressed physician, it can be helpful to ask about the physician's change in mood or behavior. While denial is a common feature of substance abuse, once a physician acknowledges a problem, doctors show better rates of recovery than the general population.[lxxxix]

ANXIETY

Physicians, along with the rest of Americans, are at high risk for anxiety disorders—anxiety is the most common mental health disorder in the United States, after all! The core dysfunction in anxiety are intrusive or perseverative thoughts which are negative and irrational, and can lead to compulsive and avoidant behaviors.

For example, if a person has a fear of elevators, the elevator is the trigger. The intrusive or wrong thought is: *"If I go in that elevator, I am going to die,"* including mental images of plummeting. Even if a person is told and knows logically that the odds of dying from an elevator failure are 1 in 10 billion (really, I looked it up), they continue to persevere on the thought that they are going to die if they get on an elevator. This thought causes intense distress and leads to an avoidant action—to take the stairs. Taking the stairs leads to a sense of relief, which reinforces the avoidant behavior. The next day, the person completely bypasses the trigger (elevator) and goes right to the stairs, feeding the avoidant behavior.

TRIGGER	→	INTRUSIVE THOUGHT	→	ANXIETY/ DISTRESS	→	ACTION	→	RELIEF
(elevator)		(*"I'm going to die"*)		(*feels bad*)		(take stairs)		(reinforces)

If you work on the 50th floor of a high-rise building and must be at work early, taking the stairs every day becomes dysfunctional—you can see that this is going to eventually become a problem.

Anxiety itself can be real. In other words, if you are driving on an icy road and you are driving more cautiously, your anxiety serves the function of self-preservation. The key distinguishing feature is whether anxiety thoughts are causing an impairment in your ability to function.

PSYCHOLOGY TIP

Anxiety is a normal emotion that serves the function of self-preservation. It is when the worry thoughts impair one's ability to function that we consider anxiety to become problematic.

When anxiety thoughts are irrational, they are not based on facts. Recognizing this inconsistency doesn't help us—it actually increases our distress: *"What is wrong with me that I'm afraid of an elevator when I know that my chances of dying are infinitesimal?"*

They key to coping with anxiety is being aware of intrusive thinking, using cognitive reframing as discussed in chapter 2 and for serious obsessions and phobias, a technique called *"exposure and response prevention (ERP),"* which is best done with a trained psychologist.

Rather than feeding the intrusive thought by performing the compulsive action it demands, ERP helps you to choose not to do a compulsive behavior while maintaining a level of distress caused by the stimulus. This can be extremely difficult in the beginning—sometimes patients with severe phobias and anxieties feel like they are going to *"go crazy,"* but if you don't give in and allow yourself to continue to experience the negative feelings, the level of distress will eventually fade. This is partly because it is impossible for your body to maintain such a high level of distress for very long.

It's sort of like putting your finger in a glass of ice water. If you remove it from the water the instant it starts to hurt (avoidance/compulsion), then let it warm up and repeat, it will continue to hurt over and over. However, if you leave it in the water and tolerate the pain for a little while, eventually the finger becomes numb and no longer hurts (habituates).

ROCK STAR ACTIVITY

Journaling worry thoughts

One way to help with anxiety is to journal your worry thoughts. When you have a worry thought, write it down. Then, identify the potential causes or triggers of the thought.

Worry thought	Level of distress 0-10	Triggering Event

ROCK STAR ACTIVITY

Anxiety journal

If you have been experiencing anxiety, complete this journal for seven days in a row. Then practice cognitive reframing of anxiety thoughts as explained in chapter 2 for one month. Now, repeat the journal exercise for seven days. Note your progress.

Each evening before you go to bed, rate the following:

1. Your AVERAGE level of anxiety on a scale of 0-10 (0 is none, 10 is as much as you can imagine)
2. Your MAXIMUM level of anxiety on a scale of 0-10
3. What percentage of the day you felt worried

Pre-assessment

Date	Average anxiety	Maximum anxiety	% of day worried

Post-assessment (after practicing cognitive reframing for 1 month)

Date	Average anxiety	Maximum anxiety	% of day worried

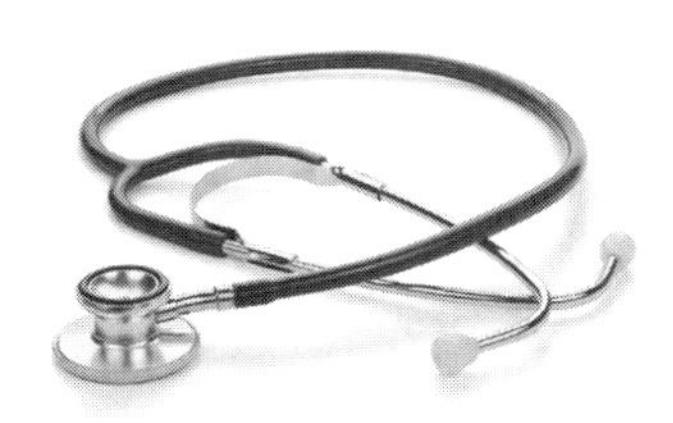

CHAPTER FOURTEEN

MENTAL HEALTH—SURVIVAL OF THE FITTEST: RESPONDING TO EXTERNAL FORCES

Mental strain often comes from external forces, and physicians may be particularly vulnerable unless we take steps to protect ourselves.

POST-TRAUMATIC STRESS DISORDER (PTSD)

Physicians are at an increased risk for post-traumatic stress disorder, with studies showing that about 15% of emergency room physicians have experienced PTSD,[xc] as well as 13% of medical residents (20% of the women and 9% of the men).[xci] Physicians who practice in underserved and remote areas, those involved in malpractice suits, and doctors who are indirectly exposed to trauma (such as hearing stories from their patients, or caring for trauma victims) are also at an increased risk for developing PTSD.[xcii]

Unfortunately, physicians are exposed to traumatic situations on a regular basis, such as repeated exposure to death. We may also experience vicarious trauma and intense helplessness when we can't help someone and have no choice but to move on to the next patient. Physicians are also subject to the strain of "emotional labor"—the effort required to put on a happy face despite how we feel on the inside.

The symptoms of PTSD can be extremely distressing. They include flashbacks or a reliving of the trauma over and over, as well as physical symptoms such as a racing heart, palpitations and sweating, nightmares and frightening thoughts, feeling easily startled, being tense and on edge, having difficulty sleeping, and experiencing anger and emotional outbursts.

People with PTSD often want to try to stay away from places that remind them of the experience, but this can be difficult or impossible for physicians, who must work in the very areas where they may have experienced the trauma. It may be helpful to know that smell can be a particularly strong trigger for trauma as it is the only sense that is not filtered and directly triggers the limbic system.

One way to prevent PTSD is to take the time to acknowledge the emotions that tragic events evoke in us, to talk to our peers about how we feel, and to realize that it is ok to feel sad, upset, angry, hurt—even to cry. Giving vent to our feelings rather than keeping them bottled up is necessary for our emotional health.

If you are noticing symptoms of PTSD, talk to a psychologist for specialized help. In the case of a major trauma, such as an error that resulted in the death of a patient, professional help is essential and should be undertaken immediately.

ANGER

Anger is a normal human emotion and can sometimes be beneficial—when responding to injustice, or to help you deal with a threat or a difficult situation. But uncontrolled anger can easily become a problem.

Anger often stems from frustration and the belief that one is not able to overcome a situation, particularly regarding conflict and lack of control in the workplace. This frustration can bubble over and lead to uncontrollable outbursts of anger.

CLINICAL VIGNETTE

> Dr. G worked for a health system that changed to a new electronic record system that he found a complete nightmare. He suggested improvements to make the system more user-friendly, which were rejected. He became increasingly frustrated that the system was going to cause him to make a mistake and lead to a patient error. One day he became so upset and angry that he threw a prescription pad across the room, causing a tear in his rotator cuff. A week later, when his nurse entered patient information into the wrong patient's chart, he berated her until she cried, which made him feel terrible.

To reduce feelings of anger, start by acknowledging your feelings. First, label your emotion—*"I am feeling really pissed off"*—giving it a label or name causes the amygdala to pause momentarily as it knows the emotional state of anger but not the name. Then, ask yourself *"why am I so angry?"* Is your anger justified? If so, perhaps you need to take steps to change your situation. Take some deep breaths while you mull this over, as breathing has been shown to improve feelings of anger.

Next ask yourself, how do I *want* to feel? Consider the ideal set of feelings: calm, controlled, reasonable.

And finally, ask yourself, *"What do I need to do to feel the way I want to feel?"* By asking yourself that question, you force yourself to engage your frontal lobe and to re-engage your executive functions which the limbic system had temporarily shut down. The nice thing is you don't even need to come up with the answer!

Sometimes the way that people deal with anger is by removing themselves from the situation that is causing the frustration. But this won't work if you continue to ruminate on the negative events.

Rather than dwelling on the negative feelings of anger and aggravation, focus on your *"goal"* or what you are or were trying to accomplish when you became frustrated. Think about ways that you can achieve that goal. For example, Dr. G in the vignette became angry about his bad computer system. Rather than perseverating on all the ways that the system is terrible, he could consider workarounds. Or he could start plotting an exodus from a system that prevents him from practicing medicine in line with his values.

PSYCHOLOGY TIP

Use anger as a tool—redirect your feelings towards focusing on your goal. What were you trying to accomplish when you became frustrated?

ARROGANT/ OVERASSERTIVE BEHAVIOR

Anger and frustration sometimes causes us to lash out at others, like Dr. G in the vignette above, who yelled at his nurse because of his frustration with the electronic health record. Burnout itself can also cause unwanted behaviors, with cynicism and detachment leading to the use of sarcasm and aggressive behavior.

Being rude and insulting towards colleagues and staff members rarely goes over well and can get you into trouble. This behavior is hurtful towards others and ultimately hurts you as a physician—if you keep it up, it won't be long before you are being labeled as a "disruptive" doctor and paying a visit to the Human Resources office.

The best way to manage this type of behavior is to get to the root of the problem. If you find yourself "acting out," ask yourself what is *really* triggering the behavior. This is painful, because 1) it requires you to acknowledge poor behavior, and 2) it may require you to consider making some major changes to your current situation.

But if you don't get control over your behavior, soon enough, someone else will be making those decisions for you, like sending you to anger management classes or before a review board. Better to deal with it yourself first—with a psychologist, if necessary.

How to "make up" for bad behavior

The key to resolving this issue is to *"own"* the behavior. For example, if you find yourself being rude, condescending or overassertive towards staffers, first acknowledge the offending behavior. *"Sue, I yelled at you when I saw the mistake in the computer record."* Next, state how you think it made them feel. *"That must have made you feel very uncomfortable and hurt."* Tell them that you will try not to do it again, but let them know that if you do, they should tell so that you can correct the behavior. Be vulnerable enough to give permission to correct you. *"I will try not to yell again. If I do, please remind me that I am not to yell at staff members."*

LOW SELF-CONFIDENCE

> *"Good judgment comes from experience and experience comes from bad judgment."* – Attributed to multiple sources

Sometimes the reason that we behave inappropriately is because of lack of self-confidence. We may demonstrate arrogant or overconfident behavior as a way of overcompensating for feelings of insecurity, or *"imposter syndrome."*

Women physicians in particular may experience low self-confidence with a reduced sense of personal accomplishment, or a sense that what you are doing doesn't matter, which can lead to feelings of frustration and hopelessness.

We need to remind ourselves that while we feel insecure and underconfident, our patients believe in us and trust us. The reality is that, as perfectionists, we are always striving for perfection, yet to practice medicine is ultimately to experience failure.

One way to improve self-confidence is by focusing on building our social confidence and becoming more self-aware of the reactions of those around us. When we lack self-confidence, we assume that everyone is looking at us and judging us, even if this may not actually be true. To challenge this belief, we must determine if this is actually a fact or a false preconception. We can do this by learning social awareness or by attuning ourselves to the reactions of those around us.

Developing social awareness to build self-confidence

To become more self-aware, first become more aware of others. For example, when talking with someone who becomes defensive, I must first notice that they are acting defensively (arms across chest, lips pursed). After noticing this, my next thought should be: *"Am I doing something that is causing them to be defensive?"*

I can determine that by checking my own body language to assess what signals I am sending. I may need to adjust my own social cues (perhaps sitting in a more open and accepting manner with arms open and a slight head tilt) to help improve the other person's level of comfort.

We are not inherently good at paying attention to subtle social cues and gestures—it takes training and practice. We often see only what we want to see or what we expect to see, and we miss an awful lot of what we don't want to see.

Think about it like this: when you go to a magic show, unless we know where to look for the magician's sleight of hand, we will miss the way they palm a card, or hide a coin. These objects aren't really disappearing, but because of our lack of perception, they will appear to be *"magically"* gone. Once we are shown how the magic trick actually works, suddenly everything seems obvious.

The same thing happens when we practice watching the body language and social cues of others. With practice, we can get better. A psychologist or body language expert can provide more insight into learning how to read and respond to the social cues of others. We have also included several books on body language in Appendix A.

Standing up for yourself

When we have low self-confidence, it can be hard to stand up for ourselves even when we face injustice or mistreatment. It may be very anxiety-provoking to think about speaking up to a colleague or superior—partly because, as we discussed in Chapter 3, we have been practicing wrong thinking when we imagine the scenario.

Instead of imagining your heart pounding, palms sweating, and the room staring you down as you stand up for yourself, voice squeaking, visualize yourself calm, cool, heart beating slowly, dry palms, nice deep breath as you speak in a clear, confident voice to the person who has treated you unfairly. You speak eloquently but succinctly. The person listens to you, blinks a few times, and apologizes profusely—they will correct the problem at once. You thank them briefly, turn on your heel, and walk away, feeling confident.

CLINICAL VIGNETTE

Dr. D was a new Pediatrician at a group practice. The medical director, Dr. N, also a pediatrician, did mostly administrative work but was scheduled to see patients on Fridays. On Dr. D's first week of practice, several additional patients appeared on her schedule on Friday. "*Oh, those are Dr. N's patients,*" explained the office manager. "*Sometimes he doesn't have enough time to see them because of meetings, so he re-assigns them to other doctors.*" Dr. D was surprised, as she had a full schedule, but she stayed quiet. The next week, the same thing happened. Week after week, Dr. D saw Dr. N's patients, and seethed with the injustice of it. But rather than confronting Dr. N and acknowledging her emotions, Dr. D became more and more frustrated until she had an angry outburst, leading Dr. N to label her as a "disruptive" doctor and put her on a performance improvement plan.

The reality is that most of the time simply acknowledging an injustice, rather than repressing your feelings is all that you need to do to take back control and gain confidence. Dr. D in the vignette above could have made an appointment with Dr. N, and said, calmly: "Dr. N, I see that every Friday your patients are being assigned to my schedule. I already have a full schedule and I wasn't sure if this was an oversight or an expectation that I need to accommodate." Sometimes just acknowledging when an incident first occurs can clarify that this is not simply an oversight or correct a situation before it becomes a pattern.

While we don't know how Dr. N would have responded, we do know that at least Dr. D would have had the opportunity to acknowledge her feelings rather than repressing them, which ultimately caused her more problems in the long run.

Acknowledging feelings, even when they are uncomfortable, is the first step to taking control. The more we do this, the easier it gets and the more confidence we gain. Nowhere is this truer than in the case of sexism and sexual harassment.

RESPONDING TO SEXISM AND SEXUAL HARASSMENT

Most women physicians have been sexually harassed in the workplace, including by patients.[xciii] In general, women tend to find themselves responding to sexism and sexual harassment with feelings of embarrassment, anger, and frustration.[xciv]

And although most women report that they want to confront sexism, the reality is that when it does occur, we overwhelmingly stay silent, either due to embarrassment, lack of preparation or uncertainty of how to respond or concern for how our response will be received.[xcv]

CLINICAL VIGNETTE

Dr. C called a patient to discuss his lab results. Out of the blue, he said: *"You know, if I wasn't married, we would be together."* Dr. C. was stunned. *"I felt like a deer in the headlights. I didn't know what to say, or how to respond. I just ignored the comment and asked if he had any questions about his lab results."* Unfortunately, ignoring the comment didn't work. *"Don't get so excited,"* the patient said, his voice dripping with sarcasm. The rest of the phone conversation was incredibly awkward, as Dr. C. tried to redirect the conversation back to the patient's plan of care.

Women must acknowledge that we are likely to experience sexism at some point in our training and career. Now we can formulate a strategy to respond to inappropriate comments and actions.

How to respond to sexist comments

First, be aware that studies show that women need not be afraid to *"call out"* men when they make sexist remarks. In fact, confronting sexism openly has been shown to have positive effects on relationships between men and women.[xcvi]

Always acknowledge sexist remarks, even though it may feel uncomfortable to do so. Then respond in a controlled way and continue the conversation as though the comment had no emotional impact. The simple act of repeating back the offensive sexist remark often provides enough of a buffer to allow you to think of an appropriate controlled response.

PSYCHOLOGY TIP

Always acknowledge sexist or biased remarks—don't let them slide! The more we confront bias, the more we can reduce bias in the future and the more empowered you will feel.

In the case of the vignette above, simply repeating back the patient's own words: *"You're saying that if you weren't married we would be together?"* and then responding in a calm and controlled manner: *"It's not appropriate for you to talk that way to me,"* before transitioning back to the medical conversation would have been preferable to ignoring the patient's remarks. It is also a good idea to practice feeling the actual emotional reaction that you want to have as you respond to a sexist remark or while being sexually harassed. Visualize yourself in control of the situation, responding calmly, feeling cool and collected.

The key to decreasing sexism and gender bias is acknowledging and confronting bias in a calm and controlled manner. This simple technique can reap major rewards including the potential for reduction in overall sexism.[xcvii]

PSYCHOLOGY TIP

This technique also works for other inappropriate remarks—whether they are sexist, racist, homophobic, cultural, or other forms of bias.

ROCK STAR ACTIVITY

Practice considering alternate explanations

A strategy for coping with angry thoughts is to practice cognitive reframing. If a person has made you angry, try coming up with three alternate explanations for their behavior. For example, if you are driving to work and another driver cuts you off, your first thought may be: *"What an asshole!"* Instead of going along with your first instinct, force yourself instead to come up with three alternate theories of why they acted that way:

1. He's a student learning how to drive
2. He's on his way to the ER with an emergency
3. He spilled coffee on himself and he reflexively jerked the wheel

Practice this technique whenever you see someone do something that doesn't immediately make sense to you or if the person's actions cause you to react emotionally. You can also practice this on yourself when you do something and think *"Why the heck did I do that?"*

ROCK STAR ACTIVITY

Practice responding to uncomfortable situations

Think of a time when someone made a comment to you that made you feel uncomfortable ____________________________

____

____

____

How did you feel? ___________________________________

____

____

____

Now, imagine yourself simply repeating back what they said, telling them that what they said was inappropriate, and visualize yourself being calm and in control as you do so.

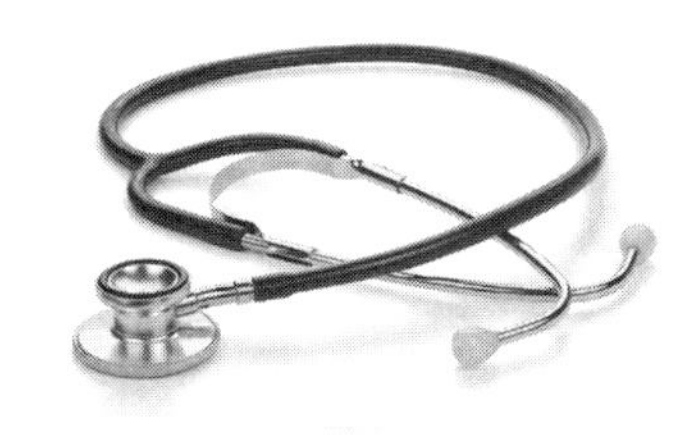

CHAPTER FIFTEEN

ADDRESSING THE MENTAL TOLL OF ILLNESS, DEATH, AND DYING

Doctors often give until it hurts. As we have discussed, we come into work when we are sick and depressed, work after hours on burdensome systems, and care for long rosters of patients with physical and mental illness. This takes a toll and can lead to something called compassion fatigue.

CLINICAL VIGNETTE

Dr. K worked in a rural underserved clinic as a National Health Service Corps Scholar. He started out with very high levels of empathy and goals of really making a difference for the community, but by the end of his first year, he found himself growing irritable and short-tempered with his patients. After hearing yet another story from a patient who didn't buy her medicine because her son stole all her money to buy drugs, he blew up: *"What's the point to this? Working with 'these people' is just an exercise in futility!"*

COPING WITH COMPASSION FATIGUE

Compassion fatigue is real, but we can take steps to prevent it from taking over by acknowledging the very human emotions that we feel in difficult situations. It helps to spend time with our colleagues talking about how we feel and to get professional help in coping before we are overwhelmed. It's also critical to remember that the physician should not be working harder than the patient—the patient is the one with the problem, after all. We must learn to set up boundaries. While acknowledging emotion is healthy, we don't want to take it home with us.

Acknowledge your own emotions

Being a physician is demanding, both physically and emotionally. If we don't learn to acknowledge and process our emotions in a healthy way, we can become psychologically damaged. In fact, studies show that the decline in empathy levels in third year medical students may be related to the sudden exposure to illness and death which often remains unexamined, ignored, and repressed.[xcviii] Rather than acknowledging the uncomfortable emotions that our training elicits, we may develop maladaptive coping techniques, like the use of black humor, cynicism, or detachment.

In fact, physicians deal with some pretty bad stuff every day. We must tell people that they have a terminal illness. We get the news that a long-time beloved patient has died. We have patients curse and berate us. We may receive a letter that we are being sued for malpractice. And the worst part is that sometimes, right after something awful happens, we may have to turn around and walk into the next room and act as if we are perfectly fine. We can't give any indication to our next patient of how we feel, no matter how much we are hurting inside. We shove our emotions down, we compartmentalize. And although we might be able to do this for a little while, eventually this type of behavior is going to cause us psychological damage if we don't deal with it properly.

Managing powerful emotions

Throughout our day, physicians probably interact with 20-30 different personality types—patients, coworkers, staff members, administrators—enough to send us through a whirlwind of emotions. But amongst those different people, there are bound to be one or two who create very powerful emotions—people who bring out your deepest anxieties, fears, or insecurities.

CLINICAL VIGNETTE

> Dr. A's mother was diagnosed with schizoaffective disorder when she was 12 years old. During her childhood, Dr. A took on many of the responsibilities of caring for her younger siblings when her mother was mentally unstable or hospitalized following suicide attempts. Dr. A's mother died while she was a medical student. Later in her years as a practicing family physician, she often found herself emotionally triggered by depressed women patients, who would make her think of her mother with great sadness.

Certain patients may often bring out negative emotions in physicians. James Groves, MD in his classic 1978 article, *"Taking Care of the Hateful Patient,"* describes feelings of *"fear, despair, and even malice"*[xcix] reported by physicians. We are often shocked and horrified to realize that we have these feelings, and experience guilt and anxiety over them. But the truth is, it's OK to have emotions. We all have them, and they are part of being human.

But we must *acknowledge* our emotional reactions. We must reflect on our feelings rather than repressing them. One way to help to understand your emotional reactions is by talking about your feelings in a safe environment—perhaps with a trusted colleague or a professional. Keep in mind that even anger and sadness can serve a function and understanding the usefulness of all our emotions can help us to thrive.

Sometimes our patients can remind us of painful experiences that we would rather not confront, particularly in the exam room. Perhaps we grew up with an alcoholic or mentally ill parent, and now we are facing a patient with similar issues who cause us to flashback to our own childhood memories. We may find ourselves avoiding these types of patients, shortening our time with them or treating them in a less personalized way.

But when we do this it causes increased distress, because we feel guilty about not providing good care. And that can lead to burnout. Instead of avoiding these patients and suppressing our emotions, we must acknowledge the feelings that these patients cause in us. By simply acknowledging *"this patient reminds me of my mom, and that hurts. I wish my mom hadn't suffered like this. I wish I hadn't suffered because my mom was sick like this."*

Other times patients may *"push"* your buttons. You may have a patient who challenges you on every single thing that you suggest. Or a patient may refuse to answer a question directly. This can cause intense frustration for the physician. The best way to address these patients is by being very direct and bringing light to the patient's trait. For example, *"I notice that every time I ask you a question, you change the subject. Why is that?"* Or *"I'm glad that you have come to me for advice. But I notice that every time I make a recommendation, you decline it. Why do you think that is?"*

DEALING WITH THE DEATH OF A PATIENT

Eventually we all face the death of a patient. The more directly we care for patients and the more responsible we feel for their outcomes, the more impact their deaths tend to have on us. When a death is unexpected, the patient is young, or we are very close to the patient, it may hit us very hard emotionally. A physician can also be particularly distressed by a patient death if we feel blamed for the outcome or if litigation is involved.

CLINICAL VIGNETTE

> Dr. B opened the newspaper to learn that her patient, a young mother, had been murdered by her husband. Over the next few days, she would hear a tragic story of domestic violence that her patient had never revealed to her. Dr. B pored over the patient's chart for signs of abuse that she may have somehow missed or clues that she could have picked up, tormented by the idea that perhaps she could have somehow done something to prevent this outcome. To make matters worse, Dr. B was the family doctor for the victim's children and parents as well and seeing them in the office over the next days to weeks caused her great grief and anguish.

Physicians who lose patients report feelings of self-doubt, failure, guilt, and powerlessness. One of our first instincts when we learn of a patient death is to worry that perhaps we missed something or somehow contributed to the patient's death: Could I have somehow prevented this outcome? We may feel a sense of failure, or a loss of control that makes us question our abilities as physicians.

Physicians also report sadness after a patient death, including experiencing insomnia and crying. Unfortunately, grief in medical training has been considered weak or unprofessional; something shameful to keep hidden away. Rather than openly expressing grief, physicians instead use the technique of compartmentalization– putting the painful emotions into a metaphorical sealed box, which we move into the attic of our mind away from everything else where we can pretend it doesn't exist.

Sometimes it is necessary to compartmentalize briefly to do our jobs. For example, if we are working in the emergency room performing on an unsuccessful cardiac resuscitation, we may not have time to process that patient's death before rushing into the next room to help a patient having a heart attack. In this case, we may have to *"box up"* the first death to focus on the second emergent situation. However, we can't leave our grief in a box indefinitely without having negative consequences.

While compartmentalizing can work for the short-term, our subconscious *does* remember that the box of emotions is still there, waiting to be opened. If we continue to ignore and repress those bad feelings, we will start to feel their psychological effects over time. This is true no matter how emotionally stable, immune, resilient, or secure you believe you are.

In addition to compartmentalizing, physicians also use other techniques to avoid our negative thoughts or emotions. One is isolation—dismissing from our consciousness any uncomfortable thoughts or feelings. Another is distraction—focusing all our energy on an alternate task to avoid thinking about grief or negative thoughts.

These techniques can become maladaptive if we use them to put up emotional barriers to prevent us from addressing our feelings, rather than engaging in healthy coping mechanisms and accepting support from others. Unexamined emotions ultimately lead to distraction, inattention, irritability, emotional exhaustion, and burnout. [c] Further, unacknowledged grief impairs physician-patient relationships and can negatively impact physicians' own personal lives.

The bottom line is that doctors must accept that death and grieving is a normal part of life. Moreover, doctors need time and space to grieve. Grieving does not have to mean staying home from work or crying for hours at a time. It can include simply acknowledging and reflecting on the emotions that a patient's death creates in you, talking about your feelings with family, friends or peers—and avoiding maladaptive techniques of isolation and distraction, including numbing yourself with drugs or alcohol.

PSYCHOLOGY TIP

Acknowledge the emotions that patient outcomes including death create in you, as a physician. Death and grieving is a normal part of life.

When a death is particularly impactful or traumatic, it may be beneficial to reach out for professional help from a bereavement counselor or psychologist for support. Sometimes taking some time off from work may be necessary to process these strong emotions.

Reach out to family members

One technique that can be very helpful when we lose a patient is to reach out to their family members. A condolence card or letter, simply expressing your sadness at the patient's passing and a few personal words about the patient can mean so much to a grieving family. When a death is sudden or unexpected, don't be afraid to pick up the phone and call the family directly to express your shock and sadness. Invite family members in to the office to talk over the situation to help them understand what may have happened medically and provide closure.

CLINICAL VIGNETTE

Dr. S, a child psychiatrist, was deeply saddened to learn that a sixteen-year old patient of hers, "Todd," had committed suicide. Although it was emotionally painful, she contacted his parents and invited them to come in to talk. On the telephone mom was open but dad was very angry in the background, questioning why Dr. S hadn't been able to help Todd. However, both parents did come in the next week to meet with Dr. S. Everyone cried, including Dr. S. All agreed that Todd had been showing signs of getting better, but had made a sudden relapse into depression, and his suicide could not have been predicted or prevented. They had tried their best.

COPING WITH DYING PATIENTS

While the death of a patient is often very hard on doctors emotionally, sometimes coping with a dying patient is even more difficult. There are several reasons. First, let's examine this statement on the view of medicine in the United States: the *"dominant unspoken philosophical basis of medical care is a form of Cartesian reductionism that views the body as a machine and medical professionals as technicians whose job is to repair that machine."*[ci] Following this model, once a patient is dying, it stands to reason that my job as a medical technician is done. The machine is irreparably broken, so I need to move on. Next patient!

But this can't be right. Because a patient is still a human being, with physical and emotional needs, even if functionally *"irreparable."* This leads to a conflict that most physicians aren't always prepared for—how do we shift gears from *"technician-healer"* to helper, comforter, and consoler? And are we able to give up our role and urge to *"do-everything"* to be able to focus on comfort without feeling as if we have given up or failed?

When faced with these many overwhelming thoughts, one defense mechanism may be a desire to withdraw or dissociate from dying patients. But our patients need us at this time in their lives possibly more than ever.

One of the most important roles that the physician can take on at end-of-life is to nurture our patients' courage by providing support and not abandoning them. We can offer them dignity and respect. Doctors can help patients to find some form of fulfillment or meaning in their lives—

even by just having patients reflect on the role that they played in their career or community, raising their family, in creativity, or by being a positive influence on another individual in their lives.[cii] Sometimes what our patients need most is simply to be there and to hold their hand when they die.

CLINICAL VIGNETTE

Dr. S, a psychologist, had worked with "TJ," an 8-year-old boy with congenital HIV-infection for many years. TJ developed cytomegalovirus of the brain, and was no longer able to eat or drink, requiring a PEG tube for feeding and a tracheostomy and mechanical respirator to breathe. TJ was suffering greatly, and he asked to be taken off the respirator and tube feeds. Dr. S spent many hours with him leading up to this, along with physicians, to ensure that TJ and his parents understood the implications. TJ had one request for Dr. S: *"I want you to be there when they turn off the machine."* To this day, this remains one of the most emotional memories for Dr. S. He was present when TJ passed away, holding his hand.

Another challenge for physicians is that working with dying patients can lead us to our own existential crisis, where we are forced to ask ourselves those very core questions:

- What is the meaning of life?
- Why do bad things happen to good people?
- And we may not be able to help but wonder: Will this horrible thing someday happen to me or someone close to me?

Perhaps one of the reasons that we try so hard to "save" our patients or that we have trouble letting go despite exhausting all reasonable interventions is because of personal struggle with these existential questions.

Again, we must acknowledge the emotions that death and dying cause us. The uncertainty, the angst, the anxiety, the not-knowing, the mere thought of our own mortality—it weighs upon our spirit, and it impacts our behavior. Many physicians find solace and comfort in seeking answers and wisdom through faith, from spiritual leaders, through prayer, from history and ancient texts. The truth is out there, I'm told.

ROCK STAR ACTIVITY

Talk to your colleagues

Schedule a regular time to meet with your colleagues to facilitate the opportunity to discuss thoughts and feelings related to negative patient outcomes.

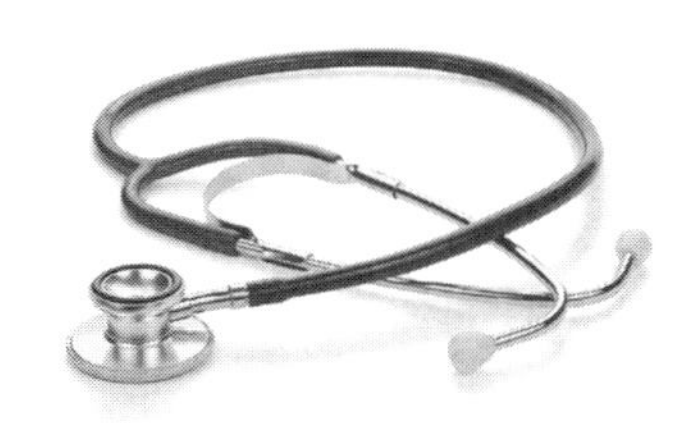

CHAPTER SIXTEEN

MENTAL HEALTH AND THE BAD OUTCOME

Physicians often live in fear of making a medical mistake. As has been pointed out (ad nauseum), doctors tend to be perfectionistic. We sacrifice ourselves to help people and we often feel guilty and anguished when something does go wrong.

The problem with worrying excessively about mistakes is that the more we try not to make a mistake, the more distracted we become. And, when we lose our focus, we increase our risk of error. For example, if you ask someone to do a puzzle without any time limit, and then you have them do a puzzle of the same difficulty with a time limit, they will perceive the second puzzle as much more difficult.

The reality is that as humans, we will err at some point in our careers. When this inevitably happens, the key is to own the mistake. Be as open and honest as possible with your patient. Don't abandon them because you feel uncomfortable and anxious. It's when we don't admit that something went wrong that patients usually feel the most discontent with their physicians.

WHAT TO DO WHEN YOU MAKE A MISTAKE

We don't necessarily have to admit wrong-doing when we acknowledge a mistake or a bad outcome. We can simply and sincerely say that we are sorry that a person is in pain or suffering or that something didn't go the way you wanted it to. We can also offer ways to make the situation better whenever possible. The good news is that, in general, communicating well with patients, including disclosure of mistakes may decrease the risk of one of our greatest fears: a malpractice lawsuit.[ciii]

Most doctors are anxious about the prospect of being sued for medical malpractice. It's a stressful experience that tends to be extremely expensive and lengthy, with the average lawsuit taking five years to resolve.[civ] Unfortunately, we have reason to be concerned, as 42% of physicians are sued at some point in their careers.[cv] The really sad part is that the legal system is neither fair nor just, as most malpractice suits are completely without merit. In fact, data shows that two-thirds of the claims are dropped, withdrawn or dismissed.[cvi]

Lawsuits are a major cause of burnout amongst physicians, and lead to emotional exhaustion, stress, depression, and personal dissatisfaction.[cvii] Being sued once also increases the risk of being sued a second time, possibly due to the adverse emotional effects that the initial lawsuit causes on the physician.[cvii]

When we do receive notice of a lawsuit or potential suit, we often respond with feelings of shock, outrage, anxiety or dread. As with other anxieties, we may find ourselves ruminating on the case and having intrusive thoughts that force their way into our minds when we are trying to focus on other tasks. We may worry about the publicity of a trial, what others will think of us, and the implications on our reputation and sense of integrity.

CLINICAL VIGNETTE

Dr. S, an experienced cardiothoracic surgeon in an affluent area was sued after the death of a public figure during open-heart surgery. During the trial the local newspaper featured the events of each day as front-page news, including scandalous allegations by the prosecution regarding the surgeon's supposed mistreatment of the patient. The trial lasted several weeks, and the articles prominently featured the prosecution's allegations and downplayed the defense's response that nothing was improper, the patient was extremely high risk with low probability of surviving any cardiac surgery regardless of the skill of the surgeon. At last the verdict was found for the defense—Dr. S was not guilty. The newspaper reported the verdict—on the back page behind the classified ads.

It is important to be aware of our thoughts, feelings, and our physical symptoms throughout the litigation process. A big part of litigation is a sense of being *"out of control,"* as we are now in unfamiliar territory in a new, adversarial relationship that is completely different from our physician's role. While our attorneys can guide us in the legal aspects, we need to talk with our family, a trusted colleague, and a psychologist to help cope with the emotions generated by this stressful situation.

PSYCHOLOGY TIP

While risk managers and lawyers will advise physicians not to talk to "anyone" about pending litigation to avoid jeopardizing their case, your psychologist is exempt from this advice. Think of your psychologist like a priest—everything you say is strictly confidential.

According to Sara Charles, MD, a psychiatrist and malpractice expert, it can help physicians involved in a lawsuit to focus their time outside of court on areas where they do have control and mastery, like spending time with family and friends, perhaps teaching in an area of expertise or working in a committee where their participation is valued.

At the same time, physicians should avoid working in practice areas that cause anxiety and feelings of loss of control during the case. Instead, focus on hobbies and exercise, take vacation, do financial planning, and other activities to take care of yourself. She also reminds us that malpractice cases are about compensation, not competence: *"Those who are sued are often the best in their field in working with sick and high-risk patients, and most physicians are eventually vindicated."*[cix]

RESPONDING TO BAD REVIEWS

One of the core causes of physician burnout is the concept of asymmetrical rewards—all the hard work and effort put into 99% of your day can completely fade away in response to one single negative response or complaint. Nothing makes this point better than patient satisfaction surveys or online patient review sites which are now a dime a dozen.

Any disgruntled patient—or even a malicious person who isn't even a real patient—can write a scathingly critical physician review, anonymously, of course. These reviews often leave a physician, particularly one who really cares about the work that he or she does, feeling blindsided, hurt, and angry. We rarely have any recourse to respond to online reviews—confidentiality laws prevent us from defending ourselves from complaints (not that our response would necessarily make a difference), and review websites generally won't remove comments, even when asked.

But what if I told you that the occasional negative patient complaint online could actually turn out to be a *good* thing for your reputation?

Guess what? It can! You see, there's this interesting little concept in psychology called *"pratfall effect."* It turns out that we like people who have a few flaws much better than we like people who seem *"perfect"* or invincible.[cx] So, if a physician has nothing but five-star reviews, they may seem intimidating and be perceived as less likeable than the doctor that has mostly five stars and one horrendous one-star review.

The other positive thing that can happen when we get a bad review is that the occasional detractor can bring out our champions. Most of the time people who really like us don't take the time to write us reviews. But when patients who like their doctor see a vicious review of a doctor that they care about, then look out! Patients will often rush to that doctor's defense, and you will then see a string of positive reviews that quickly neutralize a negative review.

Although this may happen organically, we can always improve our online reviews by asking our patients to write reviews of our practice. There is nothing wrong with this—*"the solution to pollution,"* after all, "*is dilution."* The more positive reviews that you have online, the less likely that a negative review will be noticed.

Another way to negate unwanted comments on review sites is to take control of your social media and web presence. The more web presence you have, the more likely it is that when someone searches for your name or practice, your own sites that *you control* show up ahead of doctor rating review sites.

It's much easier to do this than you might think. Start by making a Google page for yourself and for your business, as well as a Facebook page. You can add a Twitter account or Instagram if you feel ambitious. Create a website using an online service that makes it easy to do yourself (and remarkably affordable—my service costs $4 per month and I created it myself with minimal computer know-how)[cxi], or hire a professional website developer to help you. Many online websites even offer free SEO (search-engine optimization) services that allow search engines like

Google to find your website when people are searching for keywords that you have linked to your site ("family physician" or "general surgeon" for example).

How to respond to angry patients

It's best not to respond to patients when they post an angry comment about you or your practice in an online forum. But how do we approach the patient who writes an angry letter about your care?

In these cases, typically the best response is no response—at least to the patient. There is no real benefit to igniting the situation, as you won't get any sense of closure—generally the patient won't write you back or respond to your response, and so there won't be any real satisfaction. The patient has told you what they wanted to say. Your best response is to file the letter in the patient's chart and send them a formal letter terminating their relationship with the practice per your office protocol.

However, you should acknowledge your feelings—these kinds of letters hurt. Usually they involve some type of misunderstanding or confusion, but they are rarely something that the patient is willing to work on if they are firing off angry missives. Then call your therapist if you need to talk.

ROCK STAR ACTIVITY

Ask for reviews

Create a handout to give to patients asking them to leave reviews for your practice.

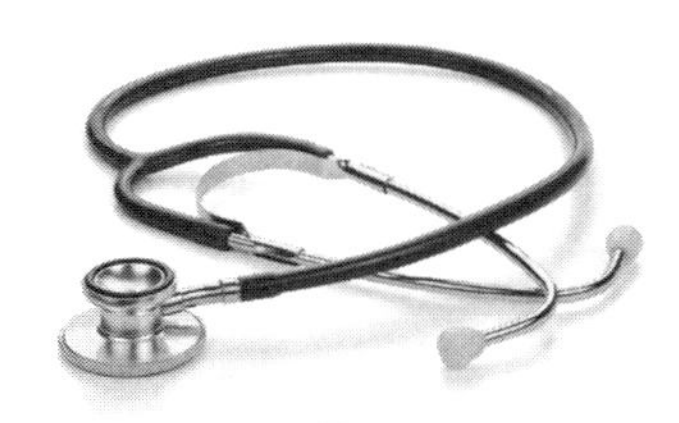

CHAPTER SEVENTEEN

USE PSYCHOLOGY TO DEVELOP HEALTHY HABITS

Doctors are notoriously bad patients. First off, we're expected never to get ill, which is completely nuts, but seems to be a common misconception. (When I had a bad cold and had to stay home from work, one of my college-educated friends said, in all seriousness, *"wait a minute, I thought doctors didn't get sick?"*)

When we do get sick, we come into work anyway. We deny, we avoid, we tough it out. We treat ourselves. We curbside consult our friends and colleagues. One in three of us has no regular source of medical care.[cxii] This is messed up.

For Pete's sake, get a regular doctor. Get a checkup. Get your pap. Get your cholesterol checked. Treat your blood pressure. Act like the mere mortal that you are. When you are sick, stay home from work. You will be surprised at how compassionate your patients will be towards you.

99% of your patients will tell you "*Don't worry about me- you just get better!*" 1% of your patients will complain and be a jerk—either don't worry about them or dismiss them from your practice. Life is too short to work when you have the flu.

And while you're at it, let's clean up some of those health habits.

USE PSYCHOLOGY TO GET A BETTER NIGHT'S SLEEP

The bottom line is that one-third of all Americans don't get enough sleep to meet their basic needs. And physicians may be even more chronically sleep deprived. In one study, 70% of doctors reported sleeping fewer than the seven hours that are considered necessary to maintain optimal work performance.[cxiii]

Doctors often fall prey to a false sense of security or belief that we can function perfectly well without adequate sleep. This partly comes from the martyrdom mentality that we develop during our training years, where running a sleep deficit almost becomes a perverse source of pride.

The reality is that physicians, like anyone, need 7-9 hours of sleep per night to function optimally,[cxiv] and even short amounts of missed sleep can negatively impact our health and work performance.

For example, just one missed night of sleep impairs cognitive and motor function to the same degree as being above the legal limit of alcohol intoxication.[cxv] In other words, you are just as likely to get into a motor vehicle accident *"driving while drowsy"* as you are driving while intoxicated. And, like the stereotypical drunk driver who feels competent to drive, we often underestimate how impaired lack of sleep makes us.

On top of the problem of impaired work quality, insufficient sleep has also been shown to cause a variety of physical conditions including obesity, diabetes, and heart disease, as well as emotional disturbances including depression, anxiety, irritability, and anger.[cxvi]

How to get enough sleep?

Environment

Setting the stage for a good night's sleep starts with creating the right environment. Your room should be as dark as possible—pitch black is better than mostly dark. Hang black-out curtains in your room, or if this isn't possible, invest in a soft, comfortable night shade to wear over your eyes while you sleep.

PSYCHOLOGY TIP

Afraid of the dark? Don't be embarrassed! Fear of the dark is a common primal instinct and can be a major cause of insomnia. In one study, up to half of the participants reported being afraid of the dark, which contributed to an increase in their levels of insomnia.[cxvii] Conventional insomnia treatment often doesn't address fear of the dark, but cognitive behavioral therapy, including exposure therapy, can be extremely helpful.

Having any light in the bedroom can cause insomnia, but blue light is the worst culprit. Blue light waves tend to suppress our brain's production of melatonin, which makes it harder to fall asleep. Cover all sources of light in the bedroom—place a small piece of electrical tape over any lights emanating from electronics, get rid of lighted alarm clocks or place them in a drawer. Put your cell phone into sleep or *"do not disturb"* mode before you get into bed.

It also helps to keep a cool bedroom. The ideal temperature for sleep has been found to be around 67 degrees Fahrenheit, with temperatures over 75 degrees impairing sleep.[cxviii] This may not be right for everyone, but generally, cooler temperatures help induce sleep. It may help to wear socks though!

Your bedroom should ideally be used only for sleep and sex. Don't watch TV in bed if you can help it—if you must, leave the bedroom lights on to dilute the flickering of the television set, which stimulates the optic nerve and makes it harder to fall asleep.

Whatever you do, don't work in bed. Reading for leisure is fine and reading on a tablet or phone doesn't seem to adversely affect sleep. Just set your phone to night mode to filter out the blue light waves.

PSYCHOLOGY TIP

Don't chart in bed!

Other tips for a good sleep environment include limiting alcohol, caffeine, and nicotine. While regular exercise helps with sleep, it should be done at least three hours before going to bed. Avoid protein-heavy meals before bedtime—in fact, a small carbohydrate meal before bed has been shown to help induce sleep.[cxix] Finally, don't drink too much fluid before bed to avoid excessive bathroom visits.

Sleep hygiene

Most of us know the basics of sleep hygiene, as we often counsel our patients on sleep problems. But it's much harder to follow our own advice when we ourselves are the patients. As you read through this section, really think about your own habits, and ask what changes you can make to your own regimen.

Developing good habits

Human beings are creatures of routine and our brains are programmed to get very good at doing the same things day in and day out. Changing up a developed routine is tough, as our brain will tend to resist any change to an established pattern. The good news is that with time and some simple techniques, we can re-train ourselves into a routine that will optimize good quality sleep.

Go to bed at the same time every night and wake up at the same time every morning.

Humans have an excellent internal clock and once we establish a routine, sleep becomes much more efficient.

The best way to train yourself to a set bedtime is to simply decide what time you are going to go to bed ahead of time. Once you have determined what time you need to go to bed to get at least 7 hours of sleep, think about how you plan to implement that decision.

Consider what time you go to bed now and determine what factors may make it difficult for you to change your current pattern. If you tend to watch TV or play games on your phone at night, it may help to plan to stop those activities at least 30 minutes before your desired bedtime to avoid the *"just one more episode"* syndrome. Remember that television shows and video games are designed to keep you engaged and make it hard for you to stop. Ending a show on a cliffhanger or moving on to the next level of a game incentivizes you to continue to the next one, and the next one… until you are hours past your desired bedtime.

How to break bad bedtime habits

Sometimes we tell ourselves that we are going to do something, but when the time comes to implement the plan, we ignore our best intentions.

To break this pattern: First *be aware* of what drives unhealthy behaviors. Ask yourself: *What function does this activity serve for me?* This is especially important for repetitive activities like playing video games or scrolling through a Facebook feed for hours at a time.

Let's use social media as an example of what drives our behaviors. Studies show that Facebook users often report an increase in ego (others are "liking" your posts), as well as decreased loneliness and increased connectedness with others.[cxx] Is it possible that your use of social media is serving a function for your psyche, such as making you feel needed or wanted, which makes it hard for you to stop even when you know you need to log off and go to bed?

Another example are video games. People joke about *"Candy Crush"* addictions. But the reality is that playing games really does boost dopamine levels in the brain, which gives us a promise of reward—and, conversely, a sense of punishment when we stop. In addition, playing games can serve as an outlet or escape from the real world for some people.[cxxi] We may play games late at night because subconsciously we dread the prospect of getting up to go to work the next day.

PSYCHOLOGY TIP

Ask yourself: What function is this negative habit/ activity serving in my life? And then: What can I do to replace it?

Simply becoming aware of our subconscious drives can help us to make the positive changes that we want to develop. Then commit to turning off the video games, computer, phone, etc. 30 minutes before you want to go to sleep.

In the morning, when you succeed, acknowledge your accomplishment by saying *"I did what I said I would do."* This will intrinsically reinforce your positive behavior.

COPING WITH INSOMNIA

Assuming your insomnia doesn't have an underlying medical cause (depression, sleep apnea, restless leg syndrome, etc.), several psychologic techniques can help you fall asleep more quickly.

First, be in a positive frame of mind. It's incredibly frustrating not to be able to fall asleep, especially when you have something important to do the next day. But instead of thinking *"I hope I don't have trouble sleeping tonight,"* you need to actively engage in positive thinking. *"I'm going to fall asleep easily tonight."*

Sleep is affected by belief more than anything else. Practice thinking differently about sleep, in order to train yourself to develop a different belief. Rather than worrying about all the bad things that will happen if you don't sleep, deliberately visualize yourself sleeping comfortably.

Create a scenario in your mind in which you are getting ready for bed, turning off the light, closing your eyes, and falling asleep. See yourself drifting off to sleep. Imagine waking up refreshed after a great night's sleep. You don't have to believe it at first. You are simply using the power of suggestion to counteract your negative beliefs. But, the more you practice envisioning this positive scene, your mind will start to believe it and you will reap the rewards.

Cognitive therapy

Falling asleep isn't a matter of learning to focus on nothing. Rather, it's hyper focusing on just one thing. That's why techniques like counting sheep actually work. The problem is that counting sheep is so boring that your mind can't help but to wander to other things.

Instead, focus on something specific. One example is to invent something in your mind. If you are a car person, invent your ideal car, making it as detailed as possible. Really visualize those details. Or pretend you can be a superhero—what powers do you want to have specifically? What does your costume look like? Or you can plan your dream wedding, down to the flower arrangements and bridesmaid dresses. The more you focus on the details, the more likely you are to fall asleep before you finish.

Still can't sleep?

This technique really works. Open your eyes and stare at a spot on the ceiling or wall for two minutes. It's ok to blink. Just focus on trying *not* to sleep. Then close your eyes and rest for thirty seconds. Repeat for another two-minute cycle. Often the act of trying NOT to fall asleep will induce sleep, and you just won't be able to keep your eyes open.

Breathing exercises

Another way to help yourself fall asleep is to perform a specific breathing exercise, advocated by Dr. Andrew Weil, called the 4-7-8 breath.[cxxii] Inhale through your nose for 4 seconds, hold your breath for 7 seconds, and exhale through your mouth for 8 seconds. Repeat this until you fall asleep. This breathing technique can also work during the day for stress, anxiety, and general relaxation.

Falling back asleep

If you wake up in the middle of the night, visualize yourself going back to sleep. Think about how you feel in the morning when you alarm first goes off and you reach for snooze, because you are sooo comfortable, you feel like you weigh about a thousand pounds, and it's the best sleep ever. Often this will lull you back to sleep.

Nightmares

Psychology offers a remarkably effective way to respond to nightmares that can elicit powerful emotions that last well into our waking hours and can make it hard to fall back asleep. In the simplest scenario, use the technique of rescripting: just rewrite the dream scenario into something positive and visualize the scene to replace the negative dream.

For example, imagine you woke up from a dream in which you were falling from a tall building. You wake up just before you hit the ground (of course), and you still feel those emotions of terror. Instead of dwelling on those bad feelings, flip the script. Close your eyes, put yourself back in the dream falling, but then suddenly, you develop superpowers and voila! You can fly. Off you go, flying up and away, no longer falling, but now in control. Imagine what it feels like to fly, so free and empowered.

Or, if you dream someone is attacking you and you wake up feeling scared and vulnerable, you can think back to that scene, but suddenly you know kung-fu and totally turn the tables. You pin down your attacker through your amazing fighting moves. Watch yourself kick some butt just like Bruce Lee and feel impressed with yourself. It's your dream, after all! Take charge!

For recurrent nightmares, you can work with a psychologist to practice nightmare exposure and rescripting, which involves deliberately eliciting or remembering the nightmare to bring up the relevant emotion. Once the emotion has arisen, you will deliberately practice visualizing a different, desired emotion and develop a new dream image that matches the desired emotion.

CLINICAL VIGNETTE

Dr. B has a recurrent nightmare that she is back working in her first clinic job. The patients are piling up; the waiting room is completely full; every exam room is occupied; the charts are stacked up on her desk, and she is getting more and more behind. But she faces one obstacle after another in her efforts to catch up. She can't find a nurse to help her, the computers won't work, and so on. She starts to get more and more frustrated and then becomes angry, becoming verbally abusive with her staff. Dr. R wakes up with physical symptoms of anxiety and anger, including a pounding heart, sweats, and rapid breathing. It feels so real that she must remind herself that she no longer works in this setting, and this situation is no longer even possible.

Many physicians report post-traumatic stress disorder type dreams, in which they relive previous stressful jobs or situations, patient deaths or traumatic situations. This often results from repressed emotions or ongoing distress that hasn't been fully acknowledged or resolved. A psychologist may be able to help.

WHAT TO DO WHEN YOU WAKE UP TIRED

If you wake up and your first thought is *"I'm so tired,"* you will need to use the power of your thinking to change to something positive. Instead, while you are still lying in bed, visualize yourself jumping up, doing something active like getting the coffee going or taking a brisk shower.

If you always tell yourself you're going to get up and exercise but never actually do it, try visualizing yourself working out. See yourself putting on tennis shoes and going for a run. Then go for the run.

Early morning is another time that taking deep breaths can help. Try a few rounds of 4-7-8 breathing to energize yourself.

The good news is that once you establish a positive sleep routine, you will wake up more and more refreshed.

PSYCHOLOGY TIPS TO INCREASE YOUR LIKELIHOOD TO EXERCISE

Why is it that as physicians we know the benefits of health diet and exercise, yet we still struggle to eat right and exercise enough? Well, psychology has something to say about that. You see, knowledge is not enough. In fact, sometimes the more we know about the health benefits or deficits of a certain behavior, the more likely we are to engage or reject that behavior. For example, studies have shown that warning labels on cigarette packages may actually increase smoking behavior.[cxxiii]

Of course, knowing that our behavior is unhealthy and continuing it leads us to feel guilty. That in turn causes us to do it more, causing a vicious cycle. Someone trying to control their diet may decide, *"I'll just eat one cookie,"* which causes them to feel guilty and results in negative self-talk *("I can't believe I just ruined my diet; I just ruined everything")* which then leads to eating the entire bag of cookies. In contrast, if they believe: *"one cookie, that's ok! I've been doing really well,"* then they will move on and stay on track.

Doctors are also quite skilled at justifying that we have no time to exercise or eat healthy—we are incredibly busy, after all! But the good news is that you don't need much time to get the health benefit from exercise. In fact, one study showed that only one minute of intense exercise can produce significant health benefits.[cxxiv] One minute! That is less time than it takes to turn on your computer.

Find something you enjoy. If you hate riding a stationary bike, even if you spend money on the latest and greatest Peloton, you won't enjoy riding it. And it will just turn into the world's most expensive clothing rack.

Incorporate activity into your schedule rather than squeezing it in. Schedule exercise time and make it part of your routine. Put your workout clothes by your bed so that you see them first thing in the morning or take your gym bag with you to work so you can change at the office and head over to exercise.

Find an exercise partner. This provides accountability and increases the likelihood that you will actually exercise regularly. Hiring a trainer can also act in a similar way, by obligating you to attend your scheduled session. Attending exercise classes or group activities may also be a way to increase accountability and provide a social reward of seeing your workout buddies.

On the other hand, it's not a great idea to advertise your plans to start an exercise routine. This can backfire, because the mere *"telling"* that you are going to do something good creates its own positive feedback in your brain and decreases the drive to actually work out.

Set realistic goals. If you tell yourself that you are going to work out five days this week, and you miss one day, now the perfectionist in you feels like a failure. Set realistic goals and become an overachiever. This reinforces your positive behavior and increases your chance of continuing.

PSYCHOLOGY TIPS FOR IMPROVING YOUR DIET

It can be tough to eat right when drug reps bring by lunch or drop off cookies or other snacks, or someone has a birthday in the office and there sits a birthday cake for the third time this week. Having healthy options available to snack on is helpful, and drug reps are often very amenable to bringing in healthier options on request. Your staff may not thank you for it, but their waistlines will!

Social occasions, like office birthdays, are associated with food. This can be difficult when we are trying to watch our weight. It can help to break the connection between socializing and food—socialize with friends at venues other than barbecues or meals, like setting up a game of tennis or meeting at the gym or for a walk.

Setting yourself up for success is critical. Minimize temptation, not only at the office, but at your home as well. Why bring home food that will only tempt you? If you really want ice cream, go out and have it at an ice cream parlor, but don't keep a gallon in your freezer. Instead, make it easy to make good choices—stock the fridge with healthy choices, like ready-to-eat salads, precut vegetables, string cheese, and yogurt.

Make sure you are getting enough sleep at night. Lack of sleep has been shown to cause changes in hormone levels in our brain, which seems to increase our intake of calories and lowers our metabolism.[cxxv] So no matter how carefully you are dieting, it is impossible to control your weight if you aren't sleeping enough hours.

Consider intermittent fasting. Intermittent fasting is a technique of reducing your caloric intake for a certain number of hours per day and has been shown to help with weight loss.[cxxvi] It can be done daily or a few days per week and has also been shown in animal studies to have a potential benefit on stress resistance, brain function, and brain aging.[cxxvii][cxxviii]

If you are struggling with weight loss, working with a psychologist may help with behavior modifications or uncovering deeper psychological causes.

CLINICAL VIGNETTE

Dr. P, an internist, was about 100 pounds overweight and reluctantly considering bariatric surgery when she started working with a psychologist. As part of her therapy, the psychologist had her make a list of the advantages and disadvantages that her weight was causing in her life. She found herself surprised to list: *"Not having to date or deal with social situations"* as an advantage to being overweight. Through work with the psychologist, she realized that she was subconsciously sabotaging her weight loss efforts because of her social anxiety, and improving this through CBT, she began to have success in losing weight.

ROCK STAR ACTIVITY

Setting health goals

Identify two health goals that you want to accomplish. Set weekly objectives for each goal. Rank your level of effort and success.

SAMPLE—Weekly Goals:

Eat healthy. "I will eat three healthy meals this week."

Ranking of EFFORT: 0 1 2 3 (4) 5

Ranking of SUCCESS: 0 (1) 2 3 4 5

Go to bed earlier. "I will go to sleep at 10 pm three nights this week."

Ranking of EFFORT: 0 1 (2) 3 4 5

Ranking of SUCCESS: 0 1 2 3 4 (5)

Weekly Goals:

___

___

___

Ranking of EFFORT: 0 1 2 3 4 5

Ranking of SUCCESS: 0 1 2 3 4 5

___

___

___

Ranking of EFFORT: 0 1 2 3 4 5

Ranking of SUCCESS: 0 1 2 3 4 5

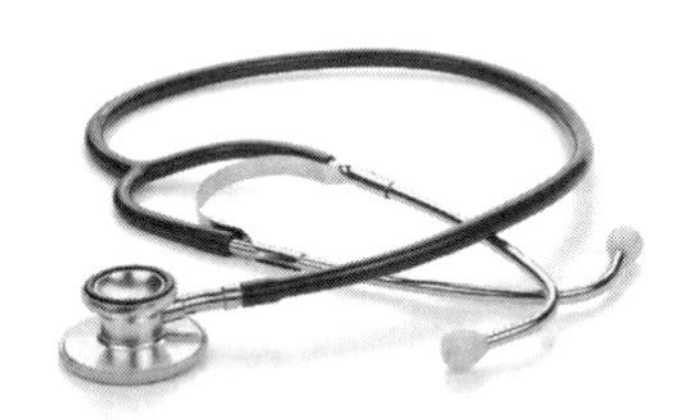

CHAPTER EIGHTEEN

USE PSYCHOLOGY TO IMPROVE FINANCIAL HEALTH

"Your 30's are for learnin' and your 40's are for earnin',"
– said no professional other than a physician

Even though physician salaries are increasing, insufficient income, inadequate savings, and debt ranked as the third leading cause of burnout in Medscape's annual physician survey in 2015.[cxxix]

So, why is it that although physicians have a relatively high income, we struggle with savings and building our retirement nest egg?

One of the biggest challenges with physician finances is that our earnings start far later than most professionals, because of the length of our education and the amount of our accumulated educational debt. We are placed at significant disadvantage with respect to both compounding interest of debt and a lack of time to allow compound interest to work on our savings.

This was demonstrated by a calculation showing that it would take the average physician 18 years to catch up to the income potential of a UPS driver who started working straight out of high school due to the advantage of compounding interest.[cxxx]

Frank Hujsa, a financial advisor in Naples, Florida who works with many physician investors, notes that doctors start out behind the eight-ball compared to other investors. The shorter time frame to build up income and retirement funds puts pressure on physicians and can sometimes lead us to make more speculative choices, like picking risky stocks or investments. *"I have noticed interesting parallels between a person's income pattern and their investment style; in the case of the physician who earns more for a shorter period, investing tends to begin later, often with higher than appropriate risk levels to 'compensate' for their late start. Ticking time bomb."*

ROCK STAR TIP

Start investing as early as possible to take advantage of time and compounding interest. Even a small amount is better than nothing.

Mr. Hujsa also points out that doctors are also easily exploited by financial advisors. *"While doctors are very intelligent and focused, they can be susceptible to overconfidence, and more trusting than the average investor. They also don't have twenty years to recover from a financial miscalculation."*

A physician's intelligence can work against us in the world of finance. Often because we know so much about our field of study, we feel that we can manage our own finances. And, indeed, we can—if we have the time and inclination to dedicate ourselves to the study of finance and investing. But a perfunctory review of investing or an assumption that just because we are smart and educated we can *"figure it out"* is just enough to get us into trouble, especially if we are working with an advisor trained to exploit us.

Physicians have some amazing qualities that make them fabulous doctors, but poor investors. First, doctors are trusting. Physicians come from a world of science, of rigorous study in which we are all educated in a standard medical curriculum, and we generally trust that our colleagues in other fields have an expert level of knowledge. Unfortunately, some financial advisors are little more than well-dressed salespeople, for whom physicians are easy prey.

ROCK STAR TIP

Use a financial advisor who is a fee-based fiduciary, which means that he or she is paid a percentage of the assets under management, as opposed to a transaction-based advisor, who is paid on commission or sales, which can create a conflict of interest.

Another quality that works great for doctors in medicine but not well in finance is that we are comfortable making quick decisions. In medicine, this helps us save lives. But in finance, this quality can lead us into dangerous territory. *"A physician's income pattern is less durable against short-term shocks,"* says adviser Frank Hujsa. So, making a snap decision and investing in a too-good-to-be-true situation can be financially devastating. Physicians may respond much too quickly to market fluctuations, putting us at risk for *"selling low and buying high."* Because of our tendencies towards quick reactions, placing financial decisions into cooler hands may be more beneficial to a physician's retirement portfolio.

Physicians also struggle with finances for many other reasons. Society sees physicians as *"rich,"* and we find ourselves expected to play the role of the wealthy doctor. After years of delayed gratification and low (or no) income, it is tempting to spend those first paychecks on a luxury car or to buy a larger-than-necessary home—especially when the bank is throwing jumbo mortgage loans at you based on your future potential income.

We also overspend out of a sense of competition—all humans have an innate competitiveness. And how much more the new physician, who has spent all of med school and residency trudging through the doctors' parking lot, filled with luxury and sports cars? We are image-conscious and we have worked hard to achieve a certain lifestyle. Spending money lavishly proves to ourselves, if not to others, that we have "made it." Buying a large home or a nice car feeds our narcissism and can also temporarily lessen our insecurity, especially for a new physician graduate who may secretly harbor feelings of imposter syndrome.

By recognizing our need for recognition and ego-gratification, we may be able to stave off the urge to spend excessively. The more confident we are with ourselves, the less we feel the need to prove it to others.

Dr. James Dahle from The White Coat Investor (2014) says that one key to financial freedom is for new physicians to try to live on a resident's salary, especially while paying down student loans.[cxxxi] As you pay down loans and your salary grows, continue to spend below your means as you save for retirement. This doesn't mean self-deprivation—we can still have a safe and decent car, and a comfortable home. But don't let your belongings own you. In other words, if you must go to work every day just to be able to pay your mortgage, your house owns you, rather than the other way around!

Remember that emotional well-being rises along with income, but only to a certain point. After an annual income of $75,000, happiness levels flatten out, and extra earnings beyond that amount don't provide much extra satisfaction.[cxxxii]

PSYCHOLOGY TIP

Money does buy happiness, but only up to a certain point (about $75,000, to be exact).

When you do spend money, studies show that you get the most bang for your buck when you spend on experiences and not on objects.[cxxxiii] While buying a sports car will make you happy in the moment, the joyful feeling doesn't last very long. On the other hand, the memories of a scuba diving trip to Tahiti will stay with you far longer.

CLINICAL VIGNETTE

Dr. T was a brand-new cardiologist at a teaching hospital. While he refused to trade in his late model pick-up truck for a shiny new sports car, he fell into a different financial pothole: a Starbucks addiction. Several times per day, Dr. T walked over to the corner coffee shop and indulged in a pricey beverage. *"At $4 per pop, 3-4 times per day, I'm spending about what I would spend on a car payment,"* he acknowledged. *"But it's my only vice, it gets me out of the office, and it's a stress reliever for me."* While Dr. T's financial advisor hates this habit and would rather see Dr. T send the $350 per month to his retirement account, Dr. T's psychologist doesn't strenuously object. *"My biggest issue is the caffeine,"* said Dr. T's psychologist. *"But overall this seems to be a reasonably psychologically healthy mechanism of stress management for Dr. T."*

Another reason that physicians get into trouble with finances is because they find the whole subject of money too daunting and choose not to think about it at all. Advisor Frank Hujsa meets physicians like this all the time. *"When I ask them about their retirement plan, they will say to me: 'I'm going to work until they carry my body out of here' or, 'my long-term care plan is my handgun,'* he says. *"Often this really means that they don't have the ability or inclination to plan."*

Dealing with finances can be anxiety-provoking and forces us to ask ourselves painful questions. Will I ever have enough money to retire? What would happen to me if I were injured or disabled? What would happen to my family if I died? Would I lose everything if I were sued for malpractice?

Rather than force ourselves to think about these issues, it sometimes feels easier to ignore them; but if we don't face them overtly, these questions linger in our subconsciousness. And they prick at us often causing us to feel financial anxiety and stress. Face uncertainty and plan for the future in order to decrease our distress and improve our psychological outlook.

PSYCHOLOGY TIP

Take the perspective and advice you give to patients about their health when it comes to finance: Don't ignore your financial health! Take proactive steps.

Another reason that many physicians fail to take steps to plan for their financial future is that it takes time, and we are busy working.

Automating our finances is an important way to minimize the time required. Set up automatic deductions from your bank account to your retirement accounts so that you don't need to think about making transfers.

Get your quarterly or biannual meetings with your financial advisor pre-scheduled in your calendar. Have your statements electronically sent to you so you don't even have to recycle huge piles of prospectuses. Make the investment process automatic and watch your money grow.

ROCK STAR ACTIVITY

Know your financial situation

Schedule a meeting with your financial advisor or at a minimum, use a personal finance software program to get a realistic idea of your financial status. Make sure that you have a retirement plan to secure your future.

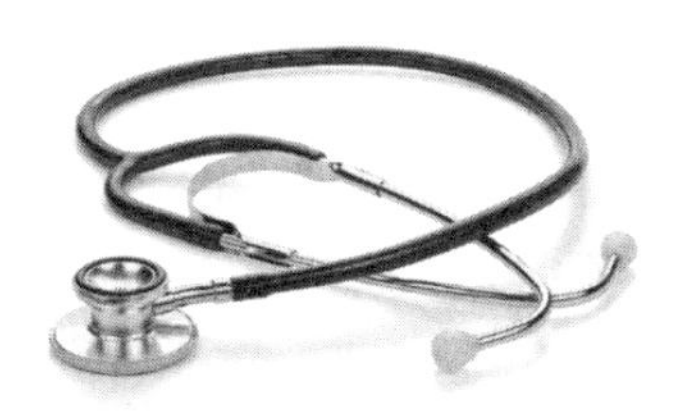

CHAPTER NINETEEN

USE PSYCHOLOGY TO TAKE BACK CONTROL

We've discussed the rates of physician burnout and the fact that most burnout comes from systemic issues. Since systemic issues are difficult, if not impossible, to change, particularly for the individual physician, most of this book has focused on taking psychological steps to cope with the stressors that the system imposes on us.

And while using psychology is a powerful tool for helping us to cope with the challenges that we face within a broken healthcare system, we are left with one important question: *Why must we continue to work in a broken system?*

I'm not talking about simply leaving the practice of medicine, taking an early retirement, or transitioning into nonclinical work. Instead, we must ask ourselves if there are any other options that let doctors practice medicine on our own terms and allow us to care for our patients without the burden of paperwork and meaningless administrative tasks.

The answer is yes.

There are alternate medical practices that absolutely allow physicians to take control of their day-to-day lives. Options include independent contract work, locum tenens, and practice ownership, including newer practice models of direct patient care or *"cash"* practices, which generally opt out of Medicare and third-party payments and contract directly with the patient for payment.

Yet, despite these career paths, most doctors continue to accept the suffering that comes from working within a broken system and we continue to show up at work day after day despite being miserable. Many of us even spend additional time trying to make the system better, such as working with our organizations on committees to improve the electronic health record or with our medical societies and political groups to lobby for changes to reimbursement. While these activities make us feel as if we are participating in being 'part of the solution,' we never have any true impact on the core defects of the system.

So why do we bother? Could it be that physicians are suffering from a sort of Stockholm syndrome?

STOCKHOLM SYNDROME

a psychological phenomenon in which hostages express empathy and have positive feelings towards their captors, sometimes to the point of defending them. These feelings are generally considered irrational considering the danger or risk endured by the victims, who essentially mistake a lack of abuse from their captors for an act of kindness.

Pamela Wible, MD an expert on physician wellness and suicide, thinks so. She is tired of hearing the term *"physician burnout,"* and argues that we should call burnout what it really is: *physician abuse.*[cxxxiv] Dr. Wible believes that the only true path towards physician wellness is to abandon the current unhealthy system in favor of a physician-friendly alternative.

One reason that physicians haven't left the system is because they don't realize they have options other than traditional W-2 employment.

For example, I was completely unaware of the concept of Direct Primary Care (DPC) until I stumbled upon a post discussing it on SERMO, a physician-only social media site. In addition, doctors may not realize the wealth of opportunities for locums or contract work right in their own backyard. At a minimum, changing from employed status to contract work allows the physician more control and flexibility. In these positions, the employer usually needs you more than you need them. For once, that puts you in the driver's seat.

ALTERNATIVES TO EMPLOYED PRACTICE

Locum tenens

You can't open a medical journal or website these days without stumbling upon an ad for a locum tenens company looking for doctors. Locum tenens is a Latin phrase that means *"to hold the place of, to substitute for."* There is a high demand for locum physicians of every specialty across the country. The highest need is in rural areas, but positions are often available right in your own backyard. Or, if you really want to get wild, international locum companies are recruiting physicians for Australia, New Zealand, Canada, and Singapore.

CLINICAL VIGNETTE

Dr. V found herself feeling burned out after 10 years of private practice. Following a divorce, she decided to take a year off to work locum tenens in New Zealand. While she ultimately ended up returning to her group practice, taking a year off did reinvigorate her enough that she felt optimistic about the future of medicine.

The advantage of locum work is freedom and flexibility, as well as the ability to avoid office politics. The tradeoff is lack of stability, unless you fall into a comfortable regular locum position that never finds a permanent doc to fill the spot. Another downside is the need to manage your own benefits, although you can handle this effectively as we will discuss later in the chapter.

Contract work

Why sign your life away as an employee of a corporation when you can be your own boss and provide independent contract work? Contract work allows you to do the type of work that you enjoy on your own terms. And many companies are willing to hire physicians as contract employees in a variety of settings—urgent care, hospital work, nursing home medical directorships, insurance record review work, research facilities, etc.

Stephanie Freeman, MD, a critical care hospital specialist, has been a contract employee for the last ten years, and now has a consulting company advising other physicians on how they can do the same. *"I jokingly say that I am 'not employable,'* says Dr. Freeman. *"I just can't dedicate my entire being to an organization and its politics and allow myself to be controlled that way."*

Dr. Freeman says that it is easy to find contract work if you know where to look. *"While some physicians can stay put and work locally, the highest need is in physician shortage areas, which means that sometimes you have to travel,"* says Dr. Freeman, who lives in a physician-saturated market, requiring her to travel for most of her assignments. *"I don't mind it. Because I'm an intensivist, I do one-week shifts, and then I come home. For ambulatory specialties with Monday through Friday work, like Family or*

Internal Medicine, physicians usually take longer assignments like two or three months at a time."

CLINICAL VIGNETTE

Dr. R, an internal medicine physician with additional certification in hospice and palliative care, worked several weekends per month moonlighting at a local hospice. Dr. R found hospice work incredibly rewarding, but what she valued the most was the ability to work on her own schedule and to disregard corporate politics completely, which she was aware of through the regular emails sent to all staff members detailing every new corporate slogan and policy change. As a contract employee, Dr. R could delete 99% of those emails without a second thought. When Dr. R left her regular job, she asked the hospice medical director for extra shifts. He was delighted, and even offered her a full-time employed position, with a generous salary and benefit package. But Dr. R knew that the joy she felt in the practice of hospice medicine would be quickly eclipsed by the pain of the bureaucracy associated with working for any organization. She elected to remain a free agent, accepting extra shifts on her terms, and retaining her control and her happiness.

Why don't more doctors consider contract work? Dr. Freeman says that many just don't know that it's an option. *"Another reason is that physicians are often uncomfortable with change," she says, "and contract work sometimes means that you have to work at different sites and adjust to different people and practice styles."*

A potential downside to working at different sites is that you may miss the camaraderie of a regular office staff and coworkers. But, on the other hand, you will meet new people. And, as a newcomer, you'll likely miss out on all the office drama.

Dr. Freeman points out that having a family isn't necessarily a deal breaker for contract and locum work. *"I've worked with many physician moms who really enjoy this type of work,"* she says. *"They either bring their family with them, sometimes with a nanny to care for the children while they are at work, or they leave the kids back at home with their spouse while they are on assignment."*

When it comes to benefits, contract employees must buy their own health insurance, but this shouldn't be a major barrier. *"While health insurance is expensive, your premiums may be tax deductible as a business expense,"* says Dr. Freeman. *"I also tell my clients that working one or two extra shifts will pay for their health insurance and then some."*

Contract physicians will also need to set up their own retirement plans—but self-employed plans can sometimes be even more favorable than traditional 401K retirement plans. *"I always advise my clients to speak to their accountant or financial planner to get a retirement plan started right away."*

PRACTICE OWNERSHIP

As the complexities of insurance reimbursement have intensified, fewer physicians are hanging a shingle and running their own medical practices. Instead, they seek the relative safety of group or hospital-employed practice. However, the tradeoff for this *"safety"* is the loss of autonomy and control, which brings an increased rate of physician burnout.

One option for physicians is to own their own medical practice, either as a solo provider or in a small group with other physicians, but selectively partner with payers to eliminate those who create the biggest burdens to the practice. For example, if an insurer repeatedly fails to pay claims, requires excessive paperwork, or is a poor payer, end your relationship with that company.

One of the most burdensome payers for many physicians are government entities like Medicare. The number of rules and regulations that physicians must follow to receive reimbursement is voluminous and ever-changing (like the 2400-page Medicare Access and CHIP Reauthorization Act of 2015, or MACRA) and requires the use of expensive electronic health records that must comply with Medicare's definition of *"Meaningful Use."*

Many physicians live in fear of a Medicare audit, with its threats of fines and penalties, which may occur even due to an honest mistake. This causes doctors to spend an inordinate amount of time double checking paperwork, clicking boxes, and confirming that coding is precise. None of this time contributes to patient care but is essential to getting paid and staying out of trouble.

But, here's the deal. No one is forcing physicians to contract with Medicare (yet). You can always decide to "opt-out" of Medicare, which means that you will no longer accept money from Medicare. If you don't take money from Medicare, you no longer must follow Medicare rules.

Physicians who formally opt out of Medicare can make private arrangements with Medicare patients allowing them to pay for services out of their own pocket. There are specific rules about how this is done, with more information available at the American Association of Physicians and Surgeons website and on the Medicare Benefit Policy Manual.

HANGING A SHINGLE, THE DIRECT CARE WAY

Even though we yearn for the freedom to run our own practice, the idea of running a conventional practice is incredibly daunting, even if we eliminate our most difficult payers as discussed above. After all, medical school offers no classes on the business aspects of medicine, and the practice management courses in residency certainly don't prepare us for the requirements of running a real practice and avoiding the pitfalls of financial ruin.

But, what if there were an easier way? What if you cut out the complicated parts of running a practice?— Eliminate all the insurance billing, as well as the complex Medicare documentation requirements, the expensive and burdensome electronic health record, and the large staff necessary to keep all that billing and coding current?

What if you just got back to what really mattered—the doctor and the patient?

What happens is an alternative practice type called Direct Patient Care. We primary care docs call it Direct Primary Care (DPC), but you can apply the concept to any physician specialist who provides medical care directly to patients.

I personally know a rheumatologist, a neuro-otolaryngologist, a gastroenterologist, and a gynecologist—all of whom function with a direct practice. In addition, loads of psychiatrists do direct care. In fact, they may have invented the very idea of a non-insurance practice, stemming from the days when most insurers wouldn't pay for mental health visits. Even surgeons and anesthesiologists are getting into the third-party payment free movement, with innovators like the Surgery Center of Oklahoma leading the way.[cxxxv]

HOW DOES DIRECT PATIENT CARE WORK?

Direct care practices eliminate third-party payers. Instead, the patient pays the doctor directly for services. Doctors don't bill any insurance companies, including Medicare and Medicaid. In Direct Primary Care (DPC), patients usually pay a monthly membership, which averages $75 per month for most practices. For specialty physicians, patients either pay a monthly membership or an a la carte cash rate for office visits, services, and procedures from a transparent price list.

At the time of this writing, there were 808 DPC practices in the United States, with many new practices on the horizon.[cxxxvi] Legislation is being drafted in many states to protect DPC practices. And several bills are pending on the federal level to promote direct care.[cxxxvii]

By eliminating the middle man—whether a private insurance company or Medicare—the physician no longer must spend 2/3 of his or her workday on deskwork, submitting data, performing mindless tasks like computerized physician order entry. Rather than spending a fortune on a bloated electronic health record, the doctor can either use a paper record or can invest in a simplified physician-friendly computerized record. The physician now has time to focus on the patient. That's the part we really enjoy and also best benefits the patient.

Compared to a traditional medical practice with its complexities of billing and coding, running a direct care practice is a whole lot simpler. And while opening a Direct care practice isn't exactly easy, it's not rocket science either. In other words, you can do it too.

GET PAST FEAR TO CHANGE YOUR LIFE

Fear is the number one reason that physicians continue to stay in a dysfunctional system despite being beaten down daily. Fear of the unknown. Fear of failure. Fear of criticism. Fear of success. Fear of having others be jealous of you. Fear of letting people down. Fear of going against the grain, and fear of what others will think of you, especially if you are a by-the-book person with a play-by-the-rules personality.

There is plenty of fear out there. Sadly, it is powerful. But there are equally powerful antidotes to fear.

The first antidote to fear is knowledge. Information, preparation, planning, resources, strategizing. Talking to others who have already been successful. Learning. Ah, we've found something that you're quite good at, haven't we?

Physicians are the ultimate problem solvers. In fact, one of the biggest sources of stress for physicians is that our brains are constantly trying to solve problems and do things better, but our administrators won't let us! *"That's not the way corporate wants us to do things..."* This creates a tremendous role strain for many doctors in the workplace.

Another antidote to fear is hope. Hope that there is another way, a better way. Hundreds of successful direct care doctors will assure you that their approach offers a better way.

And trust. Trust that you are intelligent, resourceful, and dedicated. And resilient, oh so resilient.

We yearn to do things better. And this is our chance.

Instead of just complaining and staying miserable until the day you can finally retire, take back control of your life and your profession. How? Just get past your fear.

USE PSYCHOLOGY TO GET PAST FEAR

If the book ***Dune***[cxxxviii] taught us nothing else, it's that fear is the mind-killer. But you can overcome fear. The first step to overcoming fear is to acknowledge it. Write down everything you fear. Bring your worries into full view so that you can start to analyze your concerns. Permit yourself to feel fear. After all, fear is a normal and rational emotion. You can feel it, but it doesn't have to rule you.

If you remember back to chapter 4, this is also an exercise in mindfulness—focusing on the emotion and the present state.

Now ask yourself, what is the very worst thing that could possibly happen? *"If I opened a direct care practice and it failed, what would happen?"* You would shrug your shoulders, tell yourself: well, at least I tried. And you would go back to work for another midlevel manager, no worse off than before.

"But how will I support myself financially if the practice failed?" Well, you'd probably have to cut back on expenses, take out a loan, or do some

moonlighting for a while, but would you end up living out of your car? Doubtful.

Let yourself daydream and start planning your exodus. What would your ideal medical practice look like? How would it feel to spend a year in Australia doing locum tenens, or traveling around the USA working in different places? Start reading about other doctors who made similar life changes and think about what your strategy would be.

If the idea is sounding more and more appealing, start doing some serious legwork. Gather information about your dream project, learn everything you can, and prepare yourself for a new challenge. Stay present in the moment, focusing on your goals, rather than on what might go badly and the fear of failure.

When the moment is right, or sometimes even if you're not quite ready, just take the leap. Sometimes to conquer fear, you must feel the fear and do it anyway, because it beats the alternative.

CLINICAL VIGNETTE

Dr. B had been reading about Direct Primary Care for several years. She loved the concept, but never felt quite brave enough to take the plunge. When her employer developed sudden financial problems, it felt like a sign that it was time for her to make a move. By keeping her overhead extremely low, Dr. B broke even within three months, and within a year and a half she was earning the same salary as an employed physician, but with the freedom of owning her own practice.

DEALING WITH GUILT

One of the barriers for doctors to opening an insurance-free practice is the stigma of being perceived as a *"greedy"* doctor.

CLINICAL VIGNETTE

Dr. P, a Family Physician, is in the process of converting to DPC. She feels guilty about abandoning her insurance patients after caring for them for twenty years. *"It's been huge and heartbreaking to see patients go,"* she says. She also feels anxious about *"being seen as a 'concierge' doctor"* because she fears this can be "*construed as being money-hungry and selfish. Patients can get very angry about being asked to pay more on top of [insurance] premiums."* Dr. P hopes that patients will reconcile this emotion once they understand the model and the reason that she is changing to this type of practice. *"I simply cannot keep my doors open otherwise."*

Remember that if you don't take care of yourself, you won't be able to care for anyone else—or at least not very well. So, if practicing conventional medicine has left you completely burned out, making a change may be the best way (or only way) for you to be able to continue to care for patients. Or, if the quality of your medical care is in danger of slipping due to burnout, then changing to an alternate practice can empower you to be a better doctor.

Feeling guilty about not taking insurance? Remember that direct care may allow you to treat patients who cannot afford standard health insurance or who have high deductible policies that limit their access to medical care because they can never afford the five or ten thousand dollars per year that they need to meet before their insurance starts to pay.

And, while most DPC monthly membership rates are set at very affordable levels, some DPC doctors even go the extra mile to help patients who are financially needy. Many will decrease or write-off membership payments for patients with a diagnosis of cancer. And other practices offer *"scholarships"* for patients in difficult financial circumstances.

The point is that owning your own practice without being constrained by Medicare or insurance rules enables you to help others in the way that you believe to be most effective. You can decide to forgive a membership payment or write off a bill when you want to. You can offer 10% of your memberships as scholarships for the needy. You can volunteer a few days per year at a free clinic. Or you can *"just"* provide outstanding, high quality, affordable care to your patients. That's nothing to feel guilty about!

Opting out of insurance and Medicare doesn't mean that you aren't helping people. You are just choosing a different path to helping people that is sustainable for the long term.

GET YOUR SPOUSE/ FAMILY ON BOARD

Family support (or lack thereof) can make or break your dream to leave the system for an alternate practice. Whether you are planning to cut back to part-time hours, quit your job and go locums, or open a practice on your own, this huge life change impacts not only you, but your partner and family, too.

CLINICAL VIGNETTE

Dr. S wanted to open a Direct Care practice for several years, but her husband, a non-physician, was hesitant. "*He simply didn't understand the strain of what we do—even when I came to him emotionally spent because of life-deciding decisions we all make, he just didn't get it.*" When Dr. S found herself crying as she drove to work most every day, her husband reluctantly agreed to support her dream: "*He recognized I wasn't going to be happy no matter what I did in the system.*" Dr. S now has a successful practice, but she notes that her husband still becomes angry when they discuss the transition. "*He said that though he knows it was the only option to jump when we did, he still wishes I had made my salary for another year, so we were in a better spot financially. Like most, our family made financial sacrifices, so I could open my clinic. Those sacrifices aren't over and likely won't be for a while. And these decisions will affect us long term, too, like our retirement. But ultimately, he said that if we hadn't made the leap when we did, we might not be married anymore."*

First, realize that while you may have been thinking about making this change for quite some time, this may be the first time that your partner has heard about it—at least, *really* heard about it. Maybe they have heard you talking occasionally about the concept of locum tenens or direct care, but their brains haven't registered those choices as a potential reality.

So, the first time you present the idea of making a big life change, your spouse probably won't be mentally prepared. Their first response is likely to be the normal human emotions that we associate with change: Surprise, fear, and anxiety. This is natural—they haven't had time to process the idea. So, they aren't ready for change.

The problem is that we *are* ready for change! We have been turning this concept around in our mind for months, maybe even longer, working through the emotions, reconciling them, and preparing for change. And, now when we announce our grand plan that is going to solve our problems to our spouse, we wind up with cold water in our face. This makes us feel upset and frustrated. And, in turn, when our partner becomes more anxious, the situation escalates.

The better way to plan for life changes is to involve your partner in your thought processes very early in your decision making.

ROCK START TIP

Discuss with your partner how you feel and the way you are thinking through your decisions, especially when you are considering major life changes. They need to be involved from the start.

We often try to shield or protect our partners from the negative parts of our lives or from what we perceive as unnecessary worries. We feel that it is better to avoid worrying them *"until absolutely necessary."* But when we delay sharing, we don't allow them the opportunity to think through the situation and come to terms with their emotions gradually. By trying to protect them, we may be harming them. We also aren't letting them help us by providing support and a listening ear.

If you are just starting to consider alternatives—you read about a new type of medical practice , or a you saw an ad for a locum 's opportunity and it intrigued you—and while you aren't ready to do it now, you think *maybe, just maybe, one day*, share your thinking with your spouse! Don't do it just in passing but have a real conversation.

Talk about why it interested you, and why you would try something new like this, as opposed to maintaining a traditional practice. Discuss what barriers keep you from doing it now and what would make it easier for you to do it in the future—or what worsening situation would drive you to it sooner. This will help your partner better understand your thinking and enable them to be prepared if you do decide you want to make a future change.

MAKING A MAJOR CHANGE CAN BE STRESSFUL

Although opting out of the conventional system can reduce many of the causes of physician burnout, nontraditional practices are certainly not devoid of stressors. For example, not every direct care practice thrives financially, and some take longer than others to grow and build income. It can be exhausting to work part-time moonlighting while trying to be a physician business owner. Some practices have closed or filed for bankruptcy.

Because direct care practices increase patient access via texting and email, doctors risk being overwhelmed by patient demands unless they learn to set careful boundaries. Being aware of the potential downsides to alternate practices is vital. It's not all lollipops and rainbows. That said, many doctors will agree that the worst day in direct care is better than the best day in the *'system.'*

If you do decide that making a change to your life is the right thing to do, you will want to be sure that you have support from family, friends, and maybe even a good psychologist. Because any change, even when positive, can be stressful.

In addition to that stress, you may be surprised (and a bit hurt) to find a lack of support from some of your colleagues and peers about your decision to leave the system. Unfortunately, not everyone supports doctors who are seeking alternatives to the mainstream. Remember that Stockholm syndrome we talked about? Well, prisoners who are still on death row aren't always happy to see another prisoner get a stay of execution. Also, remember that some organizations which supposedly advocate on behalf of physicians may have a vested interest in keeping us chained to our current system.

It can be helpful to connect with other physicians who have made a change or are in the process of transitioning to an alternate practice type. Virtual physician communities abound where doctors share resources and tips on every aspect of running a direct care practice. Many physicians offer free resources and mentorship. And, many physician societies have a mission of helping doctors to take back control of the practice of medicine (Appendix B).

Even if you are not ready to make a radical change right now, at least take the time to learn about the alternatives to the mainstream. Sometimes it is just encouraging to know that you have options and that, one day, you might be ready to do something different.

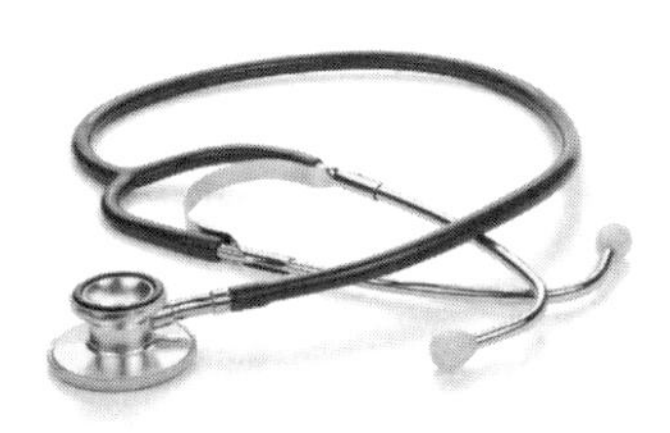

CHAPTER TWENTY

NO MATTER WHAT, NEVER GIVE UP

"If you're going through hell, keep going."
- Winston Churchill

Being a physician is more than a job. It is a calling. With that calling comes a great deal of work, stress, and sacrifice. Just because we have chosen to answer the call doesn't mean that we must do it alone.

Remember **Psychology Rule #1: The system is broken. That doesn't mean you have to be.**

You will have setbacks in your life from time to time. Sometimes you will need a little help. When this happens, psychology is there for you. It does help. We promise.

And keep in mind that, as physicians, we experience many difficult people in our lives—patients, employers, staff members, and sometimes colleagues. Like **Psychology Rule #9** says: **The people who *really* need to get help won't go. That's why the rest of us have to."**

While we can't change the way that others think and behave—we can often help ourselves interact with them more effectively by using psychologic techniques.

And, finally, no matter what, always remember this: You are a physician. That means that you are intelligent. You are resourceful. You are a problem solver. Your patients love you. You make a difference. You are resilient. You can take control of your life and your career.

As you grow in knowledge and confidence, continue to practice the techniques that we have discussed throughout the book. And, don't be afraid to reach out for extra support from your psychologist colleagues to gain more insight and tools. Because like **Psychology Rule #10** reminds us: **The better you take care of yourself, the better you can care for others.**

THE END

APPENDIX A

RECOMMENDED READING – ARTICLES

Sara C Charles MD "Coping with a medical malpractice suit." West J Med. 2001 Jan; 174(1): 55-58. https://physicianlitigationstress.org/wp-content/uploads/2014/05/Coping-with-Medical-Malpractice-Litigation.pdf

James E. Groves, MD "Taking Care of the Hateful Patient." N Engl J Med. 1978 Apr 20;298(16):883-7. http://webh01.hsl.washington.edu/reportARC/archives/hate.pdf

RECOMMENDED READING – BOOKS

Jane B. Burka PhD and Lenora M Yuen. Procrastination: Why You Do it, What to Do About It Now. DaCapo Books 2007.

James Dahle MD. The White Coat Investor. White Coat Investor LLC 2014.

Carol Dweck. Mindset: The New Psychology of Success. Random House 2006.

Mark Goulston. Just Listen: Discover the Secret to Getting Through to Absolutely Anyone. AMACOM Division American Management Association 2009.

Kelly McGonigal. The Upside of Stress. Ebury Publishing 2015.

Joe Navarro. What Every BODY is Saying: An Ex-FBI Agent's Guide to Speed-Reading People. William Morrow 2008.

Barbara Pease. The Definitive Book of Body Language: The Hidden Meaning Behind People's Gestures and Expressions. Bantam 2006.

Michael Pink. Drive: The Surprising Truth about What Motivates Us. Riverhead Books 2011.

RECOMMENDED WEBSITES

Motivational Interviewing, Bill Matulich PhD: http://www.motivationalinterviewingonline.com

Cognitive Behavioral Therapy: https://positivepsychologyprogram.com/cbt-cognitive-behavioral-therapy-techniques-worksheets/

Mindfulness: https://positivepsychologyprogram.com/mindfulness-meditation/#definition-mindfulness-meditation.

APPENDIX B

PHYSICIAN EMPOWERMENT ORGANIZATIONS

American Association of Physicians and Surgeons – https://aapsonline.org/

Benjamin Rush Institute- https://www.benjaminrushinstitute.org/

Citizens Council for Health Freedom – http://www.cchfreedom.org/

Docs4PatientCare – https://d4pcfoundation.org/

Free Market Medical Association – https://fmma.org/

MediBid: The Marketplace for Medicine – https://www.medibid.com/

Physicians Foundation – https://physiciansfoundation.org/

Surgery Center of Oklahoma – https://surgerycenterok.com/

Wedge of Health Freedom – https://jointhewedge.com/

APPENDIX C

DIRECT CARE PRACTICE RESOURCES

Douglas Farrago MD. The Official Guide to Starting Your Own Direct Primary Care Practice. Authentic Medicine 2016.

Kimberly Legg-Corba DO. Manual for Policies and Procedures for Direct Primary Care. https://dpcmanual.com/

Direct Primary Care Curriculum, Josh Umbehr, MD: https://atlas.md/dpc-curriculum/

DPC Frontier: www.DPCFrontier.com

Master Checklist, DPC Spot: https://dpcspot.com/todo.html

Pamela Wible MD http://www.idealmedicalcare.org/

AtlasMD (Electronic health record and software for Direct Care practices): https://atlas.md/

Opting out of Medicare: American Association of Physicians and Surgeons advice – https://aapsonline.org/opting-out-of-medicare-a-guide-for-physicians/

Medicare information – https://www.cms.gov/Regulations-and-Guidance/Guidance/Manuals/downloads/bp102c15.pdf

PODCASTS

http://conciergemedicineradio.com/

http://atlas.md/podcastgen/

The Direct Primary Care Podcast Show by Landon Roussel (iTunes)

The Doctor's Lounge by America's Web Radio (iTunes)

APPENDIX D:

PHYSICIAN WELLNESS PROGRAMS

This list of programs was accurate as of the time of publication and will be updated on our book website. State Physician Health Programs requiring mandatory Board of Medicine notification were not included UNLESS they also provide a separate, voluntary, confidential, non-reportable wellness program.

Alabama – Medical Association of the State of Alabama – http://www.alamedical.org/

Alaska – none at the time of publication

Arizona - Phoenix Children's Hospital – Resident Wellness Program – http://www.phoenixchildrens.org/professionals/for-students-residents/pediatric-residency-program/resident-wellness

Arkansas - Pulaski County – http://pulaskicms.org/membership/healing-the-healer-foundation/

California:

Fresno-Madera – http://www.fmms.org/programs/physician-wellness-program.aspx

Kaiser Permanente – https://scpmgphysicianwellness.kaiserpermanente.org/about-us/

Orange County Medical Association – http://www.ocma.org/for-physicians/programs/physician-wellness-program.aspx

Placer-Nevada County Medical Society – http://www.pncms.org/physician-wellness/

Colorado - Colorado Physician Health Program – https://cphp.org/

Connecticut – none at time of publication

Delaware – none at time of publication

Florida:

Collier County – http://www.ccmsonline.org/physician-wellness/

Duval County – http://www.dcmsonline.org/page/Physician_Wellness

Hillsborough County – http://hcma.net/membership-benefits/

Lee County – http://www.leecountymedicalsociety.org/en/pwp

Orange County – http://www.ocma.org/for-physicians/programs/physician-wellness-program.aspx

Palm Beach County – https://pbcms.memberclicks.net/physician-wellness-program

Tallahassee area/ Capital – https://capmed.org/resources/physician-wellness/

Georgia – none at time of publication

Hawaii – none at time of publication

Idaho - Ada County – https://www.adamedicalsociety.org/physician-vitality.html

Illinois – Chicago Latino physicians – http://www.chicagomola.com/programs/wellness-program/

Indiana – none at time of publication

Iowa - Iowa Medical Society – https://www.iowamedical.org/iowa/Iowa_Public/Resources/Center_for_Physician_Advocacy/Burnout/Iowa_Public/Issues/Burnout/Burnout.aspx?hkey=3efcfd4e-778f-422d-98f5-01975a9299b3&iSession=56cb35de70f4486199acc04e24002a2e

Kansas – Physician Wellness and Professionals Health Program – https://www.kmsonline.org/php/php-services

Kentucky - Lexington – https://www.lexingtondoctors.org/services/wellness-program/

Louisiana – Health Care Professionals Foundation of Louisiana – http://www.hpfla.org/

Maine - none at time of publication

Maryland - none at time of publication

Massachusetts - Physician Health Services – http://www.massmed.org/phshome/#.Wtt8N4jwaUk

Michigan – Wayne County – http://www.wcmssm.org/physician-wellness.html

Minnesota – Mayo Clinic – http://www.mayo.edu/research/centers-programs/program-physician-well-being/mayos-approach-physician-well-being

Mississippi - none at time of publication

Missouri - Missouri Physicians Health Program – http://www.themphp.org/

Montana – none at time of publication

Nebraska - Metro Omaha Medical Society – https://omahamedical.com/physician-burnout/provider-wellness-program/

Nevada – Washoe County – pending – http://wcmsnv.org/speak-up-there-is-help-and-support/

New Hampshire - none at time of publication

New Jersey – Mental Health Association of New Jersey (not physician specific) – https://www.mhanj.org/

New Mexico – none at time of publication

New York – Monroe County – https://www.mcms.org/Physician-Wellness-Center

North Carolina- Western Carolina Medical Society – https://www.mywcms.org/healthyhealer

North Dakota - none at time of publication

Ohio - Ohio Physicians Health Program – PHP now offering additional wellness services – https://www.ophp.org/wellnessandresiliencyprogram

Oklahoma – Oklahoma County – https://www.okcountymed.org/pwp/

Oregon:

Lane County – http://lcmedsociety.com/index.php/providerwellness/

Metropolitan Portland – https://www.msmp.org/Wellness-Program

Oregon Wellness Program- https://oregonwellnessprogram.org/

Pennsylvania- Allegheny County – https://www.acms.org/membership/physician-wellness-program/

Rhode Island - none at time of publication

South Carolina - none at time of publication

South Dakota - Avera Health Employees – https://www.avera.org/health-care-professionals/light-provider-wellness-program/light-provider-resources/

Tennessee – Chattanooga-Hamilton County Medical Society – pending

Vanderbilt University Medical Center – https://www.vumc.org/health-wellness/work-life/faculty-physician-wellness

Texas – Texas Medical Association Physician Health and Wellness – PHW help line **1-800-880-1640** https://www.texmed.org/PHW/

Travis County – http://www.tcms.com/pwp/

Utah - none at time of publication

Vermont - none at time of publication

Virginia - Medical Society of Virginia – Wellness Workshops https://www.msv.org/connections/foundation/physician-wellness

Washington -

Spokane County – http://www.spcms.org/custom2.asp?pageid=39

Washington Physicians Health Program – http://wphp.org/wellness/

West Virginia – West Virginia Medical Professionals Health Program – http://www.wvmphp.org/

Wisconsin - none at time of publication

Wyoming – Wyoming Professional Assistance Program – http://www.wpapro.org/

ACKNOWLEDGMENTS

Thank you to our amazing editor Newt Barrett for his work in editing and invaluable assistance with publication. This book would not have been possible without him.

To April Donahue and Julie Ramirez, Collier and Lee County Medical Society Executives, and Shari Skinner MD, past Lee County Medical Society President for their efforts in starting and growing our county Physician Wellness Programs to help physicians to better care for themselves and their patients.

We thank the following contributors: Stephanie Freeman MD, Frank Hujsa, Financial Advisor, Michele Parker, MD, Shane Purcell MD, and Pamela Wible, MD.

We sincerely thank the following readers for taking the time to review the manuscript and provide invaluable critique and recommendations for improvement: Niran Al-Agba MD, Poonam Bhatia MD, Deepa Burman MD, James Cohen PhD, Cheryl Iverson DO MPH, Lisa Preston-Hsu MD, and Zack Ward, EdD.

Thank you to to Dike Drummond, MD "The Happy MD" for his valuable input in titling this book and other helpful insights.

LEARN MORE ABOUT BECOMING A ROCK STAR DOCTOR!

Do you want to learn more about how to run a successful practice that delights patients while delivering financial and emotional rewards? Get ON-STAGE for clinical and professional success by following the ROCK STAR RULES in **How to Be a Rock Star Doctor: The Complete Guide to Taking Back Control of Your Life and Your Profession**. Available at Amazon in paperback and Kindle e-book edition, as well as at Barnes and Noble.

LEAVE US A REVIEW

Did you find this book helpful? Please help us to spread the word to others by dropping a review on Amazon !

SPEAKING INFORMATION

Looking for a speaker on Physician Wellness or any of the other topics you read about in this book? Contact Dr. Bernard and Dr. Cohen at our book website: www.BeARockStarDoctor.com

or at our professional websites:

www.RebekahBernard.com

www.TheCenterForPsychology.com

ENDNOTES

i http://www.physiciansfoundation.org/uploads/default/Biennial_Physician_Survey_2016.pdf

ii Cognit Ther Res. 2012 Oct 1; 36(5): 427–440.

iii *Arch Gen Psychiatry.* 2004;61(12):1208-1216. doi:10.1001/archpsyc.61.12.1208

iv American Psychologist, Vol 48(12), Dec 1993, 1181-1209

v https://doi.org/10.1371/journal.pone.0078433

vi *JAMA.* 2003;289(23):3161-3166. doi:10.1001/jama.289.23.3161

vii https://www.medscape.com/slideshow/2018-lifestyle-burnout-depression-6009235#13

viii Medscape National Physician Burnout & Depression Report 2018 Carol Peckham | January 17, 2018

ix Cognit Ther Res. 2012 Oct 1; 36(5): 427–440. Published online 2012 Jul 31

x Healthcare (Basel). 2016 Sep; 4(3): 37.Published online 2016 Jun 30

xi **DOI:** 10.1111/j.1525-1497.2000.im9908009.x

xii https://www.medscape.com/viewarticle/838437_4

xiii Maslach, C. and Jackson, S. E. (1981), The measurement of experienced burnout. J. Organiz. Behav., 2: 99-113. doi:10.1002/job.4030020205

xiv Burns, D. D. (1999). *The feeling good handbook.* New York, N.Y., U.S.A: Plume.

xv Dialogues Clin Neurosci. 2014 Mar; 16(1): 75–81.

xvi Perspectives on Psychological Science Vol 13, Issue 1, pp. 36 – 61

xvii Perspectives on Psychological Science Vol 7, Issue 4, pp. 352 – 364

xvii Journal of Consulting and Clinical Psychology, Vol 83(1), Feb 2015, 177-186 xviii https://www.today.com/health/be-thankful-science-says-gratitude-good-your-health-t58256

xix JAMA Intern Med. 2014;174(4):527-533

xx https://www.jwatch.org/fw111995/2016/09/06/half-physician-time-spent-ehrs-and-paperwork

xxi *Ann Intern Med.* 2016;165(11):753-760 http://annals.org/aim/article-abstract/2546704/allocation-physician-time-ambulatory-practice-time-motion-study-4-specialties

xxii https://mindsetonline.com/

xxiii https://www.insurancejournal.com/news/national/2011/08/19/211634.htm

xxiv https://www.psychologytoday.com/articles/200212/the-fear-success

xxv https://www.ncbi.nlm.nih.gov/pmc/articles/PMC3745291/ Clinicoecon Outcomes Res. 2013; 5: 399–406

xxvi Mayo Clin Proc. 2016 Jul;91(7):836-48

xxvii http://www.currypilot.com/newsroomstafflist/5381366-151/st-charles-scrapping-scribes-in-primary-care

xxviii https://www.aapc.com/blog/27349-confirmed-billing-provider-must-document-the-hpi/

xxix *Physician Burnout: It Just Keeps Getting Worse - Medscape - Jan 26, 2015.*

xxx http://www.danpink.com/books/drive

xxxi Mayo Clinic Proceedings , Volume 92 , Issue 1 , 129 – 146

xxxii *Arch Intern Med.* 2012; 172: 1377–1385

xxxiii The Physician Personality: Confronting Our Perfectionism and Social Isolation **Tuesday, 01 December 2009 19:00*By Lee Lipsenthal, MD - Vol. 6, No. 3. Fall, 2005***

xxxiv J Gen Intern Med. 1999 Mar; 14(3): 157–165.

xxxv *Journal of General Internal Medicine.* 1999;14(3):157-165. doi:10.1046/j.1525-1497.1999.00307.x.

xxxvi DOI: 10.1002/da.10069

xxxvii *Arch Surg.* 2011;146(2):211-217

xxxviii Academic Medicine: January 2015 – Volume 90 – Issue 1 – p 63–68

xxxix BMJ 2015;350:h706

xl D.E. Stewart, F. Ahmad, A.M. Cheung, B. Bergman, and D.L. Dell. Journal of Women's Health & Gender-Based Medicine. July 2004, 9(2): 185-190. doi:10.1089/152460900318687.

xli http://www.parenting.com/article/why-kids-need-their-dads

xlii https://www.eurekalert.org/pub_releases/2016-11/uoo-cap112316.php

xliii *Workplace Health & Safety* Vol 64, Issue 7, pp. 344 – 344

xliv Healthcare (Basel). 2016 Sep; 4(3): 37.

xlv Organizational Dynamics (2013) 42, 274 – 280

xlvi https://hbr.org/2016/07/the-data-driven-case-for-vacation

xlvii *Mayo Clin Proc.* 2016; 91: 1667–1668

xlviii J Clin Oncol. 2014 Apr 10;32(11):1127-35

xlix Am J Manag Care. 2013 Jun;19(6):509-16.

l Am J Manag Care. 2013 Jun;19(6):509-16.

li Goulston, M. (2010). Just listen: Discover the secret to getting through to absolutely anyone.

lii http://changingminds.org/explanations/theories/bystander_effect.htm

liii *Ann Intern Med.* 2016;165(11):753-760.

liv ACAD MANAGE J **October 1, 2001** vol. 44 no. 5 **1018-1027**

lv http://www.motivationalinterviewingonline.com/Welcome.html

lvi https://www.princeton.edu/~achaney/tmve/wiki100k/docs/Hanlon_s_razor.html

lvii Journal of General Internal Medicine January 1996, Volume 11, Issue 1, pp 1-8 lviii Goleman, Daniel. Emotional Intelligence. Bantam Books, 1995.

lix http://www.apa.org/monitor/oct05/mirror.aspx

lx https://www.deadiversion.usdoj.gov/pubs/brochures/drugabuser.htm

lxi Behav Processes. 2012 May; 90(1): 89–97.

lxii Pain Volume 80, Issues 1–2, 1 March 1999, Pages 1-13

lxiii https://www.samhsa.gov/data/sites/default/files/NSDUH-FFR1-2016/NSDUH-FFR1-2016.pdf

lxiv Journal of the Society of Medicine 85(10): 605–608

lxv Am J Psychiatry. 1999 Dec;156(12):1887-94

lxvi Academic Medicine 81(4): 354–373

lxvii *Canadian Medical Association Journal*. 1979;121(3):283-288.

lxviii Bright& Krahn. Current Psychiatry, 2011

lxix *JAMA*. 1977 Jan 10. 237 (2):143-5

lxx Am J Psychiatry 161:12, December 2004

lxxi *Depress Res Treat*. 2011. 2011:936327

lxxii Hawton K, Malmberg A, Simkin S. Suicide in doctors: A psychological autopsy study. Journal of Psychosomatic Research. 2004; 57:1-4

lxxiii *Arch Surg*. 2011 Jan. 146(1):54-62

lxxiv Acad Med. 2002 Sep;77(9):918-21.

lxxv http://lcmedsociety.com/index.php/providerwellness/

lxxvi Can Med Assoc J. 1979 Aug 4; 121(3): 283–288.

lxxvii Psychiatr J U Ottawa 2: 161, 1977

lxxviii https://www.psychologytoday.com/blog/anxiety-files/201111/cognitive-behavioral-therapy-proven-effectiveness

lxxix Linden DE. How psychotherapy changes the brain—the contribution of functional neuroimaging. *Mol Psychiatry.* 2006;11:528–538 lxxx Buchheim A, Viviani R, Kessler H, Kächele H, Cierpka M, Roth G, et al. (2012) Changes in Prefrontal-Limbic Function in Major Depression after 15 Months of Long-Term Psychotherapy. PLoS ONE 7(3): e33745.

lxxxi Dialogues Clin Neurosci. 2014 Mar; 16(1): 75–81.

lxxxii J Consult Clin Psychol. 1999 Dec;67(6):894-904.

lxxxiii Burnout Research Volume 1, Issue 1, June 2014, Pages 50-56

lxxxiv Myers M, Fine C. Suicide in physicians: toward prevention. *MedGenMed*. 2003 Oct 21. 5(4):11.

lxxxv Lancet. 2009 Nov 14;374(9702):1714-21. doi: 10.1016/S0140-6736(09)61424-0.

lxxxvi The American Journal of the Medical Sciences , Volume 322 , Issue 1 , 31 – 36

lxxxvii Am J Addict. 2015 Jan;24(1):30-8. doi: 10.1111/ajad.12173.

lxxxviii *JAMA*. 1992;267(17):2333-2339

lxxxix Journal of Medical Licensure and Discipline vol 93 Number 2 2007

xc https://emottawablog.com/2017/01/ptsd-for-emergency-physicians/

xci *Acad Psychiatry.* 1995;19:142-149.

xcii J Med Pract Manage. 2014 Sep-Oct;30(2):131-4.

xciii N Engl J Med 1993; 329:1936-1939December 23, 1993

xciv CMAJ. 1996 Jun 1; 154(11): 1657–1665.

xcv THE UNIVERSITY OF CENTRAL FLORIDA UNDERGRADUATE RESEARCH JOURNAL Vol. 4. Issue 2. 42–51

xcvi Journal of Experimental Social Psychology Volume 47, Issue 1, January 2011, Pages 215-220

xcvii https://www.forbes.com/sites/heidigranthalvorson/2011/09/06/3-reasons-why-it-pays-to-not-let-sexist-comments-slide/2/#722f394429a0

xcviii Academic Medicine: September 2009 – Volume 84 – Issue 9 – p 1182-1191

xcix NEJM 298 (16): 883-7, 1978 April 20

c *Arch Intern Med.* 2012;172(12):964-966

ci *Philosophy, Ethics, and Humanities in Medicine*2009**4**:11

cii Arch Intern Med. 2012 Oct 22;172(19):1501-5

ciii https://www.nytimes.com/2015/06/02/upshot/to-be-sued-less-doctors-should-talk-to-patients-more.html

civ Studdert DM, Mello MM, Gawande AA, et al. Claims, errors, and compensation payments in medical malpractice litigation. N Engl J Med. 2006;354:2024–203

cv Kane CK, ed. Policy research perspectives: medical liability claim frequency: a 2007-2008 snapshot of physicians. American Medical Association. 2010

cvi Guardado JR. Professional liability insurance indemnity and expenses, claim adjudication, and policy limits. 2000-2009. Policy Research Perspectives No. 2010-2 website

cvii Journal of the American College of Surgeons , Volume 213 , Issue 5 , 657 – 667

cviii https://physicianlitigationstress.org/identifying-and-managing-stress/burnout-malpractice-litigation/

cix West J Med. 2001 Jan; 174(1): 55–58.

cx https://blog.bufferapp.com/6-powerful-psychological-effects-that-explain-how-humans-tick

cxi Rebekahbernard.com (wix.com)

cxii *Arch Intern Med.* 2000 Nov 27. 160(21):3209-14.

cxiii https://www.sciencedaily.com/releases/2008/03/080304075723.htm

sciv https://aasm.org/resources/pdf/pressroom/adult-sleep-duration-consensus.pdf

cxv Occup Environ Med. 2000 Oct; 57(10): 649–655. doi: 10.1136/oem.57.10.649

cxvi https://www.ncbi.nlm.nih.gov/books/NBK19961/

cxvii http://healthland.time.com/2012/06/11/cant-sleep-you-may-be-afraid-of-the-dark/#ixzz24x5rCyIC

cxviii Onen SH, Onen F, Bailly D, Parquet P. Prevention and treatment of sleep disorders through regulation of sleeping habits. Presse Med.1994; Mar 12; 23(10): 485-9.

cxix https://www.psychologytoday.com/blog/the-antidepressant-diet/201411/chasing-away-insomnia-bowl-oatmeal

cxx http://www.apa.org/monitor/2013/03/cover-facebook.aspx

cxxi http://www.psychologyofgames.com/2010/07/the-psychology-of-immersion-in-video-games/

cxxii https://www.drweil.com/videos-features/videos/the-4-7-8-breath-health-benefits-demonstration/

cxxiii *Communication Research* Vol 44, Issue 3, pp. 416 – 436

cxiv *PLOS ONE*, 2016; 11 (4): e0154075

cxxv Curr Opin Clin Nutr Metab Care. 2011 Jul; 14(4): 402–412.

cxxvi *Nutrition Journ*al201211:98

cxxvii PNAS 2003 May, 100 (10) 6216-6220

cxxviii Ageing Research Reviews Volume 5, Issue 3, August 2006, Pages 332-353

cxxix *Physician Burnout: It Just Keeps Getting Worse - Medscape - Jan 26, 2015.*

cxxx http://www.er-doctor.com/doctor_income.html

cxxxi https://www.whitecoatinvestor.com/

cxxxii PNAS 2010 September, 107 (38) 16489-16493

cxxxiii The Journal of Positive Psychology, 9:4, 322-334

cxxxiv http://www.idealmedicalcare.org/blog/physician-burnout-is-physician-abuse/

cxxxv https://surgerycenterok.com/

cxxxvi https://www.dpcare.org/

cxxxvii http://www.dpcfrontier.com/blog/2018/2/9/legislative-update

cxxxviii Herbert, Frank. Dune. Chilton 1965.